Faye Koch

OSTEOPOROSIS

Your Head Start on the Prevention
& Treatment of Brittle Bones

DAVID F. FARDON, M.D.

Illustrations by Mitzi Dishman

D1087055

THE BODY PRESS
A division of Price Stern Sloan, Inc.
360 North La Cienega
Los Angeles, California 90048

This work is dedicated to
Judy, Leona, and Dorothy.
May they break no bones.

Published by The Body Press
A division of Price Stern Sloan, Inc.
360 North La Cienega
Los Angeles, California 90048

© 1985, 1987 by David F. Fardon, M.D.
Illustrations © 1985, 1987 by Mitzi Dishman
Designed by Jack Meserole
Published by arrangement with Macmillan Publishing Company

All rights reserved. No part of this work may be reproduced or transmitted
in any form by any means, electronic or mechanical, including photocopy-
ing and recording, or by any information-storage or retrieval system,
without written permission from the Publisher, except in the case of brief
quotations embodied in critical articles or reviews.

Library of Congress Cataloging-in-Publication Data

Fardon, David F.
  Osteoporosis : your head start on the prevention and treatment of brittle
bones.

  Reprint. Originally published: New York : Macmillan Pub. Co., c1985.
  Includes index.
  1. Osteoporosis—Prevention. 2. Women—Health and hygiene.
I. Title. [DNLM: 1. Fractures—prevention & control—popular
works. 2. Osteoporosis—prevention & control—popular works.
WE 250 F221o]
RC931.O73F37   1987   616.7'1   87-815
ISBN 0-89586-560-2 (pbk.)

Printed in the United States of America

10 9 8 7 6 5 4 3 2

Contents

Acknowledgments

This book is derived from the inspirations and labors of countless people whose contributions to scientific literature provide the substance of what is written here. Their courage to approach the unknown and to bare their findings to public scrutiny has endowed us with an incredibly rich fund of information. I simply have tried to organize and translate that information. I am humbly grateful to those who have provided it.

I owe personal thanks to two people who very much belong in the group acknowledged for their public contributions. Henry J. Montoye, Ph.D., included me on a research team that studied the effects of exercise on bone density and has provided me with much information on that subject. Albert W. Diddle, M.D., has been a friend and adviser and has offered me valuable suggestions about preparation of the portions of the manuscript that deal with hormones.

The superb physicians with whom I practice at the Knoxville Orthopedic Clinic, the employees of the clinic, and the staff of the Knoxville Back Care Center have provided an atmosphere in which innovative concepts can be introduced into a traditional, patient-oriented medical practice. I hope and trust that the theme of devotion to patient care prevalent at the clinic carries over onto these pages.

My wife, Judy, has contributed to this work in many ways. Her sensitivity to human needs inspired the scope of the contents and her sensitivity to my needs kept me going through this project. She provided considerable help and advice with preparation of the manuscript. Our children, Zach, Josh, Amee, and Alex, were patient with my obsession to complete this book and inspired me by their own accomplishments. Alex contributed criticism of the manuscript and was particularly diligent at ferreting out errors.

My secretary, Faye Houston, made substantial contributions to the preparation of this work. More than that, her dedication and good humor have been inspirational.

The illustrations were prepared and patiently revised by Mitzi Dishman. Glenda Clark, St. Mary's Medical Center medical librarian, and the staff of the Preston Library of the University of Tennessee Memorial Hospital helped secure many reference materials.

By training and experience I am a physician. Writing and publishing books were alien to me. Entry into that world has been eased by Bob Leggett and Dick Penner, whose advice and encouragement got me started; by David and Nancy Selby, whose enthusiasm for my earlier works stimulated me to keep going; by Richard Curtis, my agent; and by Alexia Dorszynski, Jill Herbers, and the editorial staff at Macmillan.

Most of all, I wish to acknowledge my patients with osteoporosis. I see them everywhere and their suffering has created a sense of urgency about completing this work. Bless their hearts.

This book is not intended as a substitute for medical advice from physicians. The reader should regularly consult a physician in matters relating to his or her health and particularly in respect to any symptoms that may require diagnosis or medical attention.

Preface to the
Paperback Edition

In the short time since I completed this book, some important changes have occurred. Medical sciences move—seldom smoothly or in a straight line—but nonetheless forward. There has been a wonderful arousal of public concern about osteoporosis and with it, false starts, errors, controversy and substantial progress.

Happily, what has occurred refines but does not alter the facts in the book. The amazing recent surge in public awareness has, in a much shorter time than I had expected, made osteoporosis into a household word. Virtually all major American newspapers and television networks have run features about osteoporosis. Congress has even designated a week in May as Osteoporosis Week.

Public interest stimulates research. That much is good. Public interest also creates merchandising opportunity. That can be good and bad.

The calcium pill and the dairy industries have, with huge advertising budgets, presented the public with information about osteoporosis. Their campaigns will help a lot of people, but there is a danger.

We all would like to think of osteoporosis as an easy problem with an easy solution. Wouldn't it be nice if osteoporosis were a simple calcium-deficiency disease preventable or treatable by ingesting calcium. It would be nice, but it isn't true. Broadcasters and journalists, because they need to capture the public interest with brief and dramatic presentations, have contributed to that illusion. Unfortunately, the truth is that calcium deficiency is but a small piece in a very complex puzzle.

Public concern about bone health has created other marketing opportunities. For example, after the Food and Drug Administration approved calcitonin as a treatment for osteoporosis, a drug company sponsored a campaign for physicians to train patients to give themselves regular injections of calcitonin, much in the way that diabetics give themselves insulin shots. Also, a nationwide chain of walk-in osteoporosis clinics opened, financed by revenue from photodensitometry tests.

Public information has been offered with less blatant merchandizing appeals. The American Academy of Orthopedic Surgeons published a brochure to inform patients about osteoporosis. Many prestigious hospitals and clinics have expanded their osteoporosis services so they are now more available to the public.

Parallel to public education, physicians have intensified efforts to educate one another. Osteoporosis is no longer a topic exclusive to the meetings of researchers with technical interests. It is now a common topic at meetings for physicians and other health-care providers from many specialties. Osteoporosis was the topic of the *New England Journal of Medicine's* featured review article, written for the June 26, 1986, issue by Drs. Riggs and Melton of the Mayo Clinic.

In spite of increased knowledge, *the incidence of osteoporotic fractures may have increased,* especially in men. New figures also show that the rate of osteoporotic hip fractures in women begins to rise before the age of menopause. The estimated annual cost of osteoporosis in the U.S., according to Riggs and Melton, is about six billion dollars.

Therefore, I wish to bring the reader up to date on recent events concerning osteoporosis. These recent events fall into two categories. The first involves controversy over screening methods used to detect osteoporosis. The second involves new questions regarding the effectiveness and potential side effects of different treatments: calcium supplements, fluoride supplements, estrogen therapy, calcitonin, and exercise. Necessarily, some of the concepts mentioned in this preface are technical and will be understood better after reading the book.

For patient care and for research, a means of determining the degree of osteoporosis and measuring improvement or deterioration is essential.

Controversy over the best means to do this exists in two arenas: in the staid, ivied towers of research and in a merchandizing sphere repugnant to many physicians.

Single photon densitometry, which is explained in Chapter 1, was first used to measure bone density in the forearm. Because it is safe, simple, and reasonably inexpensive, entrepreneurs marketed the idea with walk-in clinics that provided densitometry as a screening procedure for all women. Meanwhile, researchers began to question the value of single photon densitometry in assessing and predicting the course of osteoporosis, and began to extol the virtues of alternatives. The issue has been discussed emotionally in public and among health-care professionals. Both sides were represented in letters in the April 25, 1986, *Journal of the American Medical Association*. A Senate subcommittee was even asked to make an inquiry. The issue is unsettled, but the majority of clinicians agree that single photon densitometry is inadequate as an isolated test.

Dual absorption densitometry, now available in more centers, provides data that may predict hip and spine fractures better. Modifications of CT scans do the same, and CT scans are more available and less expensive than they used to be. The relative merits of these three types of screening procedures have been debated with much the same emotional rhetoric that once characterized the controversy over estrogens. Dual photon densitometry and CT scanning seem to have more scientific support, but still fall short of the kind of low-risk, cheap, available, precise, and accurate test needed to guide treatment of osteoporosis.

Almost everyone has learned that calcium deficiency may contribute to osteoporosis. The flames of public enthusiasm for calcium have been fanned by reports that calcium may reduce the risks of colon cancer and high blood pressure. While there may be some truth in such claims, we should also remember that calcium has been advocated for many things over many years (in fact, was prescribed as treatment for tuberculosis in 1800). Too, it was not so long ago that ulcer patients taking excessive calcium antacids became very ill from "milk alkali syndrome."

Reports that older people absorb less calcium and that subtle changes in Vitamin D metabolism may cause decreased calcium absorption call attention to our ignorance of calcium metabolism, our ignorance of physiologic functions in the elderly, and the need for long-term studies to answer related questions.

Reliance on calcium carbonate as a supplement also has been challenged by a study that showed that many patients with reduced stomach acid don't absorb calcium carbonate. They may need to take it with acid food or switch to calcium citrate.

Manufacturers of some vitamin/mineral supplements and some antacids have changed the contents of their products to provide more calcium or to eliminate aluminum. Consumers must check labels because brand names may remain the same while formulas change.

The National Institute on Aging, through Baltimore's Gerontology Research Center and other agencies, is collecting data that should lead to better recommendations about daily food allowances, normal laboratory values, and unique drug responses among older people.

The embittered debate over estrogen hormones died down because of clear evidence that estrogens at menopause delay bone loss. The estrogen argument, on a more dignified scientific plane, is now about potential side effects.

In the same issue of the *New England Journal of Medicine* (October 24, 1985), two separate studies were reported; one (the Framingham Study) concluded that estrogens increased risks of cardiovascular disease and another (the Harvard Nurses Study) concluded that estrogens decreased such risks. This paradox stimulated several letters attempting to explain the discrepancy. An editorial reply stated that scientific truth is a chimera and that we must accept the merits of both studies.

Meanwhile, the search continues for safer methods. New tests may help identify who needs which kinds of estrogens and who may have which side effects. Estrogen, when given through the skin, avoids the "first pass" through the liver, a passage that may affect some of the cardiovascular actions of estrogens. This is a subject of important new research, but as yet it has uncertain practical consequences. New studies have established further that smoking decreases effectiveness and increases risks of estrogen therapy.

Calcitonin has been shown to be a safe drug. Increase in total body calcium after taking calcitonin is the benefit stressed by the manufacturer and cited by the FDA in its approval of the drug for use in osteoporosis. Data to show that calcitonin prevents fractures are scanty. Researchers point to the problem of "escape," the tendency for benefits to disappear shortly after an initial favorable response. One report stated that a group of people with osteoporosis actually had high calcitonin levels, so would not likely benefit from more calcitonin.

Theoretically, calcitonin would be most effective for people who have a "high turnover" type of osteoporosis, the same type most protected by estrogens. It may be that those individuals who cannot take estrogens should take calcitonin. A great deal must be learned before the proper role, if any, of calcitonin is known.

More data have documented the favorable effects of fluorides on bones of the extremities as well as on those of the spine. The FDA's reasons for not endorsing fluoride therapy remain those discussed in this book; convenient dosages will continue to be absent from pharmacies until adequate studies are completed. While mysteries remain about why some patients respond and others do not, the safety and effectiveness for many look good in reported studies.

Recent articles about exercise reinforce the contentions that weight-bearing stress and heavy muscular effort lead to increased bone density. There are conflicting opinions about whether prolonged running damages joints, the preponderance of evidence being that such exercises will increase bone density without causing arthritis in previously healthy joints.

As often in medicine, progress produces more questions than answers. In the brief time since first publication of this book, at least some of the questions have become clearer.

Doctors need to know simple ways to identify various types of osteoporosis. They need better ways to predict and monitor severity—to settle the questions about what density measurement is best and to find blood tests that are precise, accurate, sensitive, and inexpensive. They must learn to apply measurements to treatment decisions—to know who needs which treatment, at what age, in what dose, and for how long. Simultaneously, we must search for drugs that provide more positive effects on bone strength with fewer drawbacks. All of this must be done, mindful of the fact that the bone that breaks from osteoporosis does so as a result of lifelong effects on bone health, so understanding must come from very long-range planning and study.

While many of the above needs will be supplied by scientists and health-care professionals, the public must also respond. Interest in osteoporosis must be sustained.

Public understanding must mature. We have to accept that osteoporosis is not a simple calcium-deficiency cured by pills. It is a complex disease about which we need more information and a more intelligent understanding of how to apply the very useful information we already have. We must support scientific efforts to gain new knowledge and learn to be intelligent consumers of the provisions of current knowledge.

I believe this book stimulates public efforts to cure osteoporosis and am grateful to The Body Press for making it accessible to more people by issuing this paperback edition. I hope that it will contribute to the realization of Drs. Riggs and Melton's conclusion that " . . . it is reasonable to hope that this formidable disease can be brought under control within the coming decade."

Introduction

WOULDN'T you think that the name of a disease that affects half the women over forty-five years of age would be a household word? Osteoporosis, the name of this disease, should have become part of our everyday vocabulary long ago, but perhaps the complex, medical sound of the word has delayed public understanding. The broken hips and wrists, as well as the shortened, hunched, painful spines, caused by this disease are all too familiar in our society.

Only in the past few years have popular magazines begun to feature articles about osteoporosis. In many of these articles, the word itself has been avoided in favor of less-imposing but less-accurate terms such as "brittle bones" or "porous bones." However, there is much more to the story of why this common and devastating disease has remained so unpublicized than its six-syllable name.

The movements to protect the rights of women and the elderly have called attention to the problems created by osteoporosis. Eight times as many women as men suffer from the complications of this disease. The back pain, stooped shoulders, loss of height, and broken hips, wrists, and other bones caused by osteoporosis occur increasingly with age. So, even though some men suffer equally devastating effects and even though some of the habits of early life may predispose bones to break, the enormous health problems caused by osteoporosis usually affect older women.

Many medical subjects are introduced by a description of the disease as it was in ancient times, but this is not the case with osteoporosis. Hippocrates does not mention it. Of course, the average life expectancy of a woman during his time was about thirty. By the time America was discovered, most women lived to about the age of forty. In 1923, the U.S. National Center for Health Statistics reported the average woman lived to be fifty-eight and a half. Now the average American woman lives to be seventy-eight. Osteoporosis worsens after menopause, and since women who live past menopause now live an average life of eighty-four years, they spend a third of their years after menopause.

Since 1900 the number of Americans over the age of sixty-five has quadrupled. There are about 35 million Americans over sixty. There are 22 million women over fifty-five, the age when most women are past menopause. Menopause may occur in many women at an earlier age, for a variety of reasons—the most common one is hysterectomy, 650,000 of which are performed in the United States each year. Thirty percent of those hysterectomies include removal of the ovaries, which inevitably results in a drop in estrogen output with the onset of menopause and loss of bone strength.

Statistics about the incidence of osteoporosis are difficult to interpret because the condition is hard to define precisely. Loss of bone strength is part of the normal human aging process, so there is an understandable reluctance to consider everyone a victim of osteoporosis. The border between normal, age-related loss of bone mass and excessive loss is not well delineated.

Every year at least a million Americans break bones that would not have broken had they not been weakened by osteoporosis. Everyone agrees that such people should be considered to have osteoporosis; everyone also agrees that such people also had osteoporosis on the day before they broke the bones. It is hard to estimate the number of people with skeletons so weakened by osteoporosis that their bones are just waiting to break from some trivial injury.

Each year almost two hundred thousand people in the United States break their hips. The chances of breaking a hip at age seventy are fifty times as high as at age forty. The chances of breaking a hip are ten times as high for a woman as for a man.

Complications from hip fractures are the leading cause of accidental death among the elderly. But are these fractures really from accidents? Did the fall cause the fracture or the fracture cause the fall? Rarely does the accident occur with sufficient force to break a strong bone. Besides the considerable threat to life, hip fractures cause terrible suffering, result in hospital costs of a billion dollars a year, and too often permanently diminish the quality of life.

Broken wrists are among the most common injuries requiring medical attention. When people fall, they try to protect themselves with their outstretched hands; if the force of the fall is great enough, the wrist breaks. That much is common to all ages. Until the age of forty-five, the number of wrist fractures in women is about the same as in men; after forty-five, the incidence is ten times as high in women. A German surgeon named Paul Bruns was one of the first to observe that wrist fractures occurred more often among older women. He claimed in 1882 that women broke their wrists more often because they tripped over their long skirts. We know better now.

Loss of height and a humpbacked, round-shouldered posture are so common among elderly white women that they are accepted as normal. Whoever thought of Whistler's mother as having a disease called osteoporosis? Some loss of height over a lifetime is normal to both sexes: it results from the drying of the intervertebral discs. However, this does not explain the dramatic changes in dress length to which many older women must adjust when their heights decrease.

The loss of three to eight inches in height over a few years is not normal. It results from compression fractures of the spinal vertebrae—individual bones in the spine are compressed like so many crushed shredded-wheat biscuits. This does not happen to normal bone unless it is subject to great force caused by an extraordinarily violent accident; it happens to osteoporotic bone as the result of the simple stresses of standing or the physical efforts of everyday life. The vertebrae crush more toward the front, resulting in a forward curve of the spine and humped shoulders.

Osteoporosis is much more common among whites than blacks: fair-skinned, light-haired people of northern European heritage have the highest incidence of osteoporotic fractures. By the age of sixty-five, about one in four white women have spinal fractures that can be seen on X rays. The sedentary life of the well-to-do may also contribute to bone weakening. The humped back of the elderly, affluent white woman has thus come to be called a "dowager's hump."

Sir Astley Cooper, a British surgeon, wrote in 1824 that the skeleton seemed to become more fragile with age. Wilhelm Roentgen, a German physicist, received the first Nobel Prize for his discovery of X rays in 1896. Discussions of fractures in weakened bones began to appear in German medical literature in the 1920s. In 1940 at a meeting of the Association of American Physicians, Boston endocrinologist Fuller Albright explained to his colleagues that normal bone constantly breaks down and reforms. He said that osteoporosis may result from either excessive breakdown or inadequate reformation. Albright said that osteoporosis, the common variety of weakened bones he saw in elderly women, seemed to occur because new bone didn't form fast enough to keep pace with resorption of old bone. Osteoporosis resulted from calcium loss and decrease in estrogen at menopause. The paper Albright published in 1941 in the *Jour-*

nal of the American Medical Association was entitled "Post-menopausal Osteoporosis."

Fuller Albright said most of the important things we know about osteoporosis today. Since he had an outspoken distrust of statistics, much of what he said can be taken only as the wisdom of an astute observer; some of his conclusions have proven to be untrue or remain controversial. His lack of statistical proof and his few mistakes help to explain the great delay from the time of scientific recognition until general public understanding of this problem, but they do not explain the professional community's delay in recognizing the importance of the problem.

I learned about osteoporosis in medical school in the early 1960s, but at that time it was not regarded as a pressing health care problem or as an intellectually stimulating research topic. The attitude is well exemplified by the opening sentence of an article written by Yale professor Dr. M. L. Ricatelli in 1962 in the *Journal of the American Geriatric Society:* "Osteoporosis is such a common condition that comparatively little attention is paid to it."

By the early 1960s the era of antibiotics was firmly established. The time when a president's son might die from a minor skin infection, as Calvin Coolidge's did, and when pneumonia was a highly lethal illness and syphilis and tuberculosis were medically uncontrollable cripplers, seemed to have passed. So too had the hysteria of polio epidemics. It was a time when more attention could be turned to chronic illness, but the attention turned more slowly to gradually progressive, less-dramatic problems like osteoporosis than it did to cancer and heart disease.

One reason osteoporosis was slow to receive attention was the lack of public demand. The energy behind efforts to protect the rights of women and the elderly was just gathering force in the 1960s. Information about the seriousness of osteoporosis was not, and still is not, readily available to the public. Research funding and financial support of health care projects for osteoporosis have been slow and inadequate.

Cancer and heart disease cause dramatic changes in the human anatomy, changes that made profound impressions on us as young medical students studying pathology. Fragile bones do not have the same effect. Because very ordinary problems, such as osteoporosis and its complications, are not emphasized in teaching institutions, medical students and residents do not appreciate the impact of those problems on individuals and upon society. They are eager for the satisfaction that results from treatment they have given. It is ultimately satisfying to watch a patient recover from heart failure because of medicines you have prescribed, or to remove a malignant tumor from a patient on the operating table, knowing that you got it all. It is less immediately rewarding to offer advice and prescribe medicine in hopes that at some time, years later, if the patient has continued to heed that advice, she might be spared the suffering of a broken hip.

All those obstacles notwithstanding, by the mid-1960s attention began to turn to the study of osteoporosis. In 1965 representatives from six countries met in Bethesda to design a worldwide epidemiologic study of osteoporosis. The conference was sponsored by the World Health Organization and the National Institutes of Health. Although important information resulted from the study, it is more important as a landmark of recognition of the problem.

Recognition by small research teams often predates understanding by clinicians. As a resident in orthopedic surgery in the late 1960s, I knew that patients broke wrists, spines, hips, and other bones because of osteoporosis. I knew there had been controversy about treatment with hormones and other drugs, and that the questions about the value of such treatments were unanswered. However, since I was learning how to fix osteoporotic bones and have them heal with a good success rate, I didn't think much about preventing fractures.

When I entered private practice in the early 1970s, I found the orthopedic wards of the hospital filled with motorcyclists and other daredevils hanging in traction, athletes recovering from knee surgery, and middle-aged workers receiving therapy for back-aches. Among these patients there were always little old ladies recovering from fractures, but they were sweet to talk to and easy to treat: their presence did not dominate the ambience of the orthopedic floor.

Over the past decade, fracture surgery has vastly shortened hospital stays for victims of high-speed violence; arthroscopic surgery has transformed most athletic knee operations into out-patient procedures; and room costs have become so high that very few patients with backaches are treated in the hospital. All the while, the general population of postmenopausal women has grown. Now orthopedic rounds consist of walking down the halls past one after another little, old, white woman. Each one is hunched over, hopping along on her walker to protect a broken hip. She strains to look up and say hello. In the rooms there are even more thin-skinned, fair-haired women unable to get out of bed because of back pain from recent spinal fractures. Or per-haps they are lying in bed with a recently broken wrist or ankle elevated.

Since the general public and the medical profession have in-creasingly recognized that osteoporosis is an important health problem, and since the complications of osteoporosis have come to dominate more and more of my hospital practice, I have reas-sessed my attitudes and practices regarding the disease. That led to the writing of this book. As a practicing physician, I find my interest piqued more by solutions than by problems; happily, I have discovered that there are solutions to osteoporosis. Some of these solutions have been there all along, some are new, and some are on the way.

In 1978, I worked with a team of University of Wisconsin exercise physiologists studying a distinctive group of people, all participants in the National Seniors Clay Court Tennis Cham-pionships. These tennis players were unique: they were elderly people who exercised regularly and vigorously. They were es-pecially noteworthy as experimental subjects because they had a built-in control—we did not have to compare them to other groups or other individuals. Since tennis is mostly a one-armed sport, we compared the exercised tennis arm to the inactive arm. We measured bone density and thickness, as well as muscle mass. We found, as everyone knows, that exercised muscles are larger than unexercised muscles; we also found, as the physiologists had predicted, that exercise makes bones bigger and stronger.

Exercise is one solution to osteoporosis. It is a partial solution, to be sure; there are many unknowns about how much exercise, what kind of exercise, and under what circumstances exercise prevents osteoporosis. Those details are among the remaining controversies, but it is clear that exercise is an important part of the solution. One aim of this book is to explain how and why that is true.

Hormones may also protect people from osteoporosis. Albright said that in 1940, and doctors have been arguing about it ever since. There are pros and cons to taking hormones. A *Prevention* magazine article in August 1983 concluded that the bad outweighs the good in hormone therapy. Such a generalization must be balanced against extremes of the other viewpoint, such as revealed in the address given by a University of California professor of medicine, in which he compared opponents of hormone therapy to the doctors who thwarted Ignaz Semmelweiss' attempts in 1847 to convince his colleagues to wash their hands between obstetrical cases. There are enough trustworthy, understandable data available to help lay people in making an informed decision about hormone therapy. This book provides that information without the rhetoric.

The hormone that has received the most attention in the treatment of osteoporosis is estrogen. Other hormones, such as calcitonin, progesterone, androgens (the so-called male hormones), and the body-building "anabolic steroids," all may have some value in treatment. Although there is much yet to be learned about them, there is much already known that is understandable and important to decisions about how to treat osteoporosis.

It is hard to decide whether the risks of treatment are worth the potential benefits unless you know the risks of no treatment. Some people are much more likely than others to suffer the complications of osteoporosis. Statistical bets about risk are based upon such factors as heredity, body build, and sex. You can improve the accuracy of your guess by adding medical information available from your doctor. Also, since osteoporosis may be caused by certain diseases or drugs, it can be prevented by medical attention to such underlying problems. This book provides you with the information needed to make those judgments and data about the help that may be available.

There is no doubt that proper nutrition helps to prevent osteoporosis. There is an amazing amount of controversy about what should or should not be done about diet and about vitamin and mineral supplements. Of course, there is ample room for new information from reliable research, but there is already useful information. Unfortunately, much of the good information is obscured by commercialism and the hype of enthusiasts. Some people overdo dietary supplements to the detriment of their pocketbooks, if not their health; most people are turned off by the hard sell of the enthusiasts and assume that their regular diet is enough. However, the regular American diet is not enough. There is a great need for people to improve their eating habits. This book presents diet and diet supplement information related to the problem of osteoporosis.

Calcium and fluoride supplements require particular attention. Few Americans receive enough calcium in their diets to protect them from osteoporosis. Commonly quoted recommended daily allowances of calcium do not keep up with calcium loss under many of life's circumstances. Several recent reports suggest that people with osteoporosis who take fluoride in much higher doses than those added to drinking water to prevent dental cavities may experience some restoration of lost bone. Some physicians have endorsed fluoride treatments with much the same enthusiasm that others have shown for hormone treatments.

Not all osteoporosis can be prevented. People who have already lost a substantial amount of bone may not be able to regain it. However, many broken bones can be prevented even under those circumstances by the use of aids and techniques to protect one from injury.

When a bone *does* break, it is important to understand the particular fracture, its treatment, and what to expect from it. Osteoporosis fractures are treatable: they do heal. Do not lose hope if you break your hip or your spine. It should make you angry; it might have been prevented. You should become concerned enough to make sure it doesn't happen again. This book explains what the various osteoporotic fractures do to you, what the effects of different common treatments for them are likely to be, and how you can participate in your recovery.

Who needs to know all this and when? You do and now. You especially need this information if you are female, although men are not exempt from this problem. Even if many men escape it themselves, the women they care about may not.

You need to know all of this regardless of your age. You have a "bone personality" that determines how strong your bones will be throughout life. That personality depends partly on heredity and partly on experience. Childhood diet and exercise determine the development of bone personality, and adult experience influences the maintenance of it.

It is not too late to learn about osteoporosis if you are elderly and have already suffered fractures; it is not too early if you are just beginning to learn to take care of yourself. You need to understand osteoporosis, decide what you are going to do about it for yourself and your family, continue to practice prevention, and keep informed.

I

Who Should Worry: The Risk and Diagnosis of Osteoporosis

HOW TO RECOGNIZE OSTEOPOROSIS

It doesn't take a medical specialist to recognize a person suffering the complications of osteoporosis: you can spot such people as you walk down the street. Most often, the person you recognize will be a woman in her sixties or seventies. Her head projects out in front of her body because her back is bent forward into a hump between her shoulder blades. She looks as though she should be taller than she is; her arms are too long compared to her height, and her hemline may be too low. Her face may be alert and energetic, but her body movements and muscle tone lack the vigor you would expect from looking at her face.

You can now begin to recognize people with osteoporosis in a crowd. Using those criteria, however, you will pick only those with the severe complications of osteoporosis of the spine. If you train your eye, you can begin to recognize those who have suffered complications other than severe spinal deformity.

Look at people's hands. If your hand is normal, it will angle toward the little-finger side of your forearm when you let it fall into a relaxed, flexed (bent-at-the-wrist) position. If you see someone whose hand is angled the other way, toward the thumb side of the forearm, you can be fairly sure she has osteoporosis. She has broken her wrist, the weakened bone was crushed, and it has healed in a shortened position.

Watch people walk. Not every limp is due to the residual effects of broken hips, knees, and ankles caused by osteoporosis, but many of them are. If, when you detect a limp in a woman over fifty, you bet that she has osteoporosis, you will win more bets than you lose.

Think about height. Look at photographs of people taken thirty or forty years ago and compare their height then to now. As we age, we all lose an inch or two because our discs dry up. That doesn't explain the three, four, or eight or more inches that many people lose because of crushed vertebrae caused by osteoporosis. Ask any woman over sixty how tall she was when she was thirty, and compare that with her present height. Many women think they are still five feet six inches tall, or whatever, because they have been saying so all their lives, and are shocked to find that they actually measure five feet one or two inches tall.

With just this much information, you can become adept at identifying people with osteoporosis. If you watch for them, you see them on buses, walking down the sidewalk, sitting in cafés—almost everywhere you look, though you are less likely to see them participating in sports or other physically vigorous activities. The people with osteoporosis whom you have thus far identified, however, are just those with the complications of the disease. You have seen only the permanent effects on bones that broke because they were weakened by osteoporosis. How do you know, before such complications occur, whether you or your loved ones have osteoporosis?

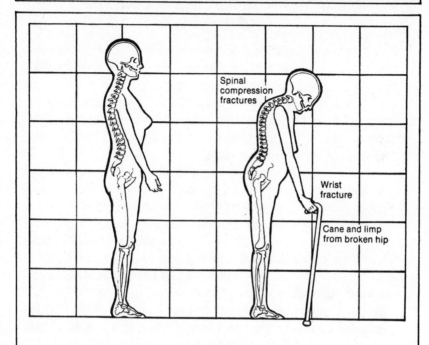

Spinal
compression
fractures

Wrist
fracture

Cane and limp
from broken hip

- Loss of height.
  Loss of trunk length relative to legs.
  Arms hang lower, fingers approach knees.

- Upper back more rounded.
  Head thrust forward.
  Abdomen protrudes.
  Ribs approach pelvis in front.

- Wrist breaks and heals with deformity.

- Cane and limp from broken hip.

HOW TO ASSESS THE RISKS OF DEVELOPING OSTEOPOROSIS

You know you have osteoporosis when you break a bone as the result of a minor injury. But do you have to wait for that? If you have had one broken bone, must you wait to see if you are at risk to have more? Fortunately, no. The diagnosis of osteoporosis can be made before fractures occur; even better, most people who are likely to get osteoporosis can identify themselves and take preventive steps.

Many diseases, drugs, and injuries cause osteoporosis, as will be discussed in Chapter 4. No one is immune to those occurrences. However, most osteoporosis is not related to any of those causes. When diseases are not related to some known cause, they are referred to as "idiopathic." While I will try to avoid unnecessary use of medical and scientific terms, it will be simpler to refer to the type of osteoporosis with no known cause, as distinguished from osteoporosis that develops from any of several identified causes, as "idiopathic osteoporosis." (Don't be intimidated by this or any other formidable-looking medical term you find here. I'll try to keep it simple, and I've provided a glossary if you have questions.) Certain people are much more prone to develop idiopathic osteoporosis than others, and those people can identify themselves.

Not all physicians agree that idiopathic osteoporosis is a single disease. Everyone's bones weaken with age, some people's more than others. Whether or not there is a clear distinction between "normal" age-related bone weakening (sometimes called osteopenia) and excessive bone weakening is controversial. Among those with excessively weak bones, there are subgroups of individuals who have certain bones that are weakest or who have characteristic ways in which their bones have weakened. These distinctions are important for research. At this time, they are not, by and large, of importance to you as you decide how to prevent osteoporosis. When we discuss the few specific problems in which such factors may have some bearing on the treatment of osteoporosis, I will call your attention to how those distinctions may be important.

Each person has bones of a certain size and strength—a bone personality. Bone personality is determined, in part, by the genes we have inherited from our parents. Each person has a unique set of genes and thus a unique capacity for bone strength. The influence of heredity on an individual can be predicted by family history and by racial background. If your parents, grandparents, aunts, or uncles showed signs of osteoporosis, your risk of developing it is higher. The highest incidence is usually found among women whose mothers showed signs of osteoporosis. It is important to distinguish the signs of osteoporosis rather than to depend upon an established diagnosis because, since popular knowledge of the disease has been lacking in the past, most older people with signs of it were unaware they had a disease by that name.

Blacks almost never develop the rapidly progressing form of idiopathic osteoporosis. They do experience slow loss of bone strength with age, but the progression is much slower than in whites. Bones weaken to the point of fracture much less often in blacks than in whites. However, blacks show the same risks for developing osteoporosis with known causes; when a black develops severe osteoporosis, there is increased concern that some disorder other than idiopathic osteoporosis may be present. Dark-skinned whites of Spanish, Italian, Greek, or Middle Eastern heritage are less likely to develop osteoporosis, while Orientals have a high incidence of osteoporosis. A high percentage of fair-skinned people whose ancestors came from northern European countries get osteoporosis.

After you assess the influences of your family and racial backgrounds, it is helpful to analyze other aspects of your genetic makeup. Certain physical characteristics are present in a high percentage of people who will develop osteoporosis.

If you are very flexible and loose-jointed, your arches fall,

and your forefoot splays out when you stand, you are at higher
risk to develop osteoporosis; so too if you have had scoliosis
(sideways curvature of the spine). People with osteoporosis usually have thin, loose skin that bruises easily and wrinkles at an
early age. If you are blond or redheaded and freckled, your risk
is higher.

If your gums tend to pull away from your teeth, you have
lost teeth early, or you have required periodontal surgery, your
risk is higher. Your dentist may have noticed on routine dental
X rays that the bone around your teeth is not as dense as it should
be; if so, your risk of having osteoporosis is high. If you are one
of the 25 million toothless Americans, and, especially if you have
had to change your dentures because they no longer fit, it is more
likely that you have osteoporosis.

What is due to heredity and what is due to environment are
subjects of ongoing controversy. With respect to bone personality, many factors that are partially due to experience may also
be partially due to genetic makeup. If your genetic makeup places
you at risk for osteoporosis, you must be especially mindful to
control your experiences to ensure that your bones stay healthy.

Sex is an obvious genetic characteristic that may have considerable environmental influence upon risk of osteoporosis.
Women develop osteoporosis more often, worse, and at earlier
ages than men. As we discuss the ways experiences influence
bone strengths, you will see that some of the reasons osteoporosis is so severe in women derive from woman's role in society. Men do develop osteoporosis. However, since they often
are genetically endowed with larger and stronger bones than
women, the complications of slowly progressive bone loss do
not appear as early. Also, the progression of bone weakness is
more gradual in men. Fractures from osteoporosis in otherwise
healthy men have been considered unusual. However, a study
of residents of Malmö, Sweden, from 1954 through 1984—during which time the hip-fracture rate increased sixfold while the

population only doubled—showed a marked increase in the occurrence of osteoporosis-related hip fractures among men.

Childhood experiences are important to bone health. Bones
grow larger and stronger until the early thirties. The size and
strength to which they grow is determined by the building materials supplied to them in the form of calcium, vitamins, and
other elements of good nutrition. Bones also grow larger and
stronger in response to the stresses of muscle pull and weight
bearing. Good nutrition and regular exercise throughout childhood build bones with reserve strength, a skeleton that will
withstand bone-weakening experiences later in life. The habits
of good nutrition and regular exercise in childhood often carry
over into adult life. If your diet and exercise habits were not
ideal during your growing years, the risk of fracture from weak
bones is high and you now need to make extra efforts to improve those habits.

In the early thirties, bones stop growing stronger and start
losing calcium and strength. Vigorous, regular exercise and certain treatments may, at times, halt that process. However, most
people slowly lose calcium and bone strength throughout life.
One index of risk for osteoporosis is age. The older you are, the
more likely it is that you have osteoporosis. Unless you take
special precautions, the longer you live the more likely you are
to develop osteoporosis. If your bones were very strong when
you began losing bone strength, and if the loss has been very
gradual, it may never matter to you that your bones are weaker
at sixty than they were at twenty. On the other hand, if your
bones were not strong to begin with, and if you have some life
experiences that cause rapid loss of bone strength, you may have
to worry about broken bones all through your mature years.

Anything that deprives you of regular exercise will weaken
your bones. Most people think they are too busy to exercise.
Until recently, many women regarded it as unfashionable to exercise vigorously, which is one reason osteoporosis is more of a

problem for women. During inactive times, when injury or illness prevents exercise, you lose bone faster. You may count up the days you have exercised vigorously, balance that total against the number of days you have been inactive, and use the result as one index of your risk for complications from osteoporosis.

Every day, your body loses calcium in urine, feces, and sweat. Women who bear children give up calcium to their children's bones during the pregnancy and for as long as they nurse. The body requires a certain level of calcium in blood and tissue fluids. Your bones act as a bank in which you may deposit and withdraw calcium. Unlike a bank, however, there are limits to how much you can deposit: the bones will only hold a certain amount. If you lose more than you take in, the calcium stored in your bones will be depleted.

Details about diet and osteoporosis are included in Chapter 6. Briefly, milk, cheese, and yogurt are foods rich in calcium compounds that can be absorbed from what you eat. Any days when you have not eaten those foods in fairly large amounts (the equivalent of four glasses of milk), you have probably lost more calcium than you have replaced. If you have had many such days, your risk of osteoporosis is increased.

Some stomach operations and intestinal diseases disturb calcium absorption. Many drugs interfere with calcium metabolism or other important aspects of bone chemistry. Those factors and other diseases that may cause osteoporosis are discussed in Chapter 4. If any of those problems apply to you, they increase your risk of osteoporosis. However, there are a few health problems, such as osteoarthritis, that actually reduce the risk of osteoporosis.

Poor health habits increase the risk of osteoporosis. Drinking alcoholic beverages too much and too often causes osteoporosis; in fact, alcoholism is probably the most common cause of osteoporosis in men under sixty. Smoking is also definitely correlated with osteoporosis. If you smoke or drink alcohol regularly, you must consider yourself at increased risk for osteoporosis.

The one poor health habit that does not cause osteoporosis is overeating. Overweight people are less likely to suffer complications from osteoporosis than thin people. There are several

TABLE I
Risk of Osteoporosis—Self-Assessment

High Risk	*Low Risk*
White or yellow race	Blacks
Females	Males
Family history of osteoporosis	No family history of osteoporosis
Northern European heritage	Mediterranean heritage
Surgical menopause	Normal menopause
Early menopause	Late menopause
Little exercise	Regular, lifelong exercise
Calcium-poor diet	Calcium-rich diet
Smoker	Nonsmoker
Regular alcoholic intake	Nondrinker
Fair skin	Dark skin
Red or blond hair	Dark hair
Loose, clear, wrinkled skin	Tough, thick skin
Loose joints and muscles	Tight joints
Flat feet	Sturdy arches
Scoliosis	No scoliosis
Small muscles	Large muscles
Underweight	Overweight
Periodontal disease	Healthy teeth and gums
Illness causing inactivity	High level of activity
Stomach and bowel disease	Normal stomach
Medicines that weaken bone	No medicine intake
Previous fractures	No fractures
Loss of height	No loss of height
Rheumatoid osteoarthritis	Definite osteoarthritis

good reasons to stay thin, but osteoporosis is not one of them. Fat may produce hormones that protect bones, and extra weight may induce some healthful stress on bones. Whatever the reasons, your risk for osteoporosis is higher if you are thin. Over 85 percent of people with symptoms of osteoporosis weigh less than one hundred forty pounds.

Although women may be born with smaller bones, exercise less, and lose more calcium and take in less than men, all those factors do not fully explain why women have so much more trouble with osteoporosis than men. Women lose bone strength faster during and after menopause. A woman whose ovaries are surgically removed before natural menopause is especially vulnerable to osteoporosis. The younger a woman is when her ovaries are removed or stop functioning, the greater is her risk. When you assess your risk for osteoporosis, it may be more important to count the number of years after menopause than to consider your age. A sixty-year-old woman whose ovaries were removed when she was twenty-five is likely to have weaker bones than a seventy-year-old woman who had a natural menopause at age fifty.

HOW YOUR DOCTOR DIAGNOSES OSTEOPOROSIS

Your doctor can do many things to determine the present condition of your bones and your risk for osteoporosis. Unfortunately, there is no single, simple, surefire test, no equivalent of a throat culture to diagnose strep throat.

As you read the following discussion of medical tests, please do not assume you need them all: you may not need any of them. Also, you do not need to memorize what the tests are and what they accomplish, and you do not even have to understand them. You already know more than most people do about osteoporosis, and if you don't want to boggle your mind with medical test information, it isn't necessary. Chances are, your doctor does not know all about all these tests either; some of them are still research tools and not practical for everyday problems.

You should read about the tests because the information is interesting: you should know, in a general way, what is available. Refer back to this discussion when specific questions arise. You may also find that some aspect of this discussion may help with a present problem, and you may want to ask your doctor about it.

BLOOD TESTS   Some routine blood tests help to uncover the instances when osteoporosis is caused by some underlying disease. The tests that determine red- and white-blood-cell counts; protein, calcium, phosphorus, and thyroid hormone levels; and serum activity of the enzyme alkaline phosphatase are the ones that help most in that way. The results of these tests are usually normal in people with uncomplicated idiopathic osteoporosis.

If the routine tests give abnormal readings, or if there are other reasons to suspect some unusual problem, your doctor may recommend more-specialized blood tests. If a vitamin-D deficiency or an overactive parathyroid gland is suspected, this can sometimes be determined from blood samples. Tests for bone marrow disease, various kinds of arthritis, and many other problems are occasionally included in an evaluation of unusual forms of osteoporosis.

With all the fuss about calcium loss and dietary calcium, it may seem strange to say that calcium levels are normal in people with osteoporosis. However, this is true: each individual's body struggles to maintain serum calcium (calcium present in circulating blood) within a narrow range. Even if total body calcium is very low, serum calcium is likely to remain within the normal range. Only when some disease throws off the control mechanism is an individual's serum calcium likely to be abnormal.

Actually, the average serum calcium of postmenopausal women is slightly higher than that of premenopausal women and women being treated with female hormones. The slight elevation of serum calcium suggests that calcium is being mobilized from the bones. Even though the statistical average of the calcium levels of postmenopausal women may be higher than average, that average is still within the normal range and most postmenopausal women have normal calcium levels. Therefore, serum calcium measurements are not useful for diagnosing osteoporosis for any one individual.

Blood tests for patients with idiopathic osteoporosis are normal under most circumstances, although the alkaline phosphatase level will be elevated briefly after a fracture has occurred.

URINE TESTS   Urine can be analyzed for the products of bone breakdown. Calcium and hydroxyproline, a component of bone protein, are the two substances most often measured. Because diet and exercise vary every day, a single measurement may not accurately reveal the usual condition. Doctors usually prefer to collect and analyze twenty-four-hour urine samples, a cumbersome and expensive process. These urine tests are used most often as before-and-after comparisons for some specific treatment of unusual cases of osteoporosis; they are not often used simply to diagnose idiopathic osteoporosis.

X RAYS   X rays help most by identifying fractures. By that time, of course, some of the damage has already occurred, but it is never too late to take steps to prevent more trouble. X rays show fractures that may have been suspected from symptoms and physical appearance. They define and localize the fractures more precisely than physical diagnosis. For example, doctors know that crush fractures of the spine that occur at the apex of the round portion of the mid-back (dorsal spine) and those that occur near where the ribs end at the junction of the mid- and lower back are often due to osteoporosis. Crush fractures from minor injury at other spinal sites suggest a cause other than idiopathic osteoporosis.

Doctors experienced in the care of fractures usually know when a fracture patient has osteoporosis. They can tell by where and how the bones break. They know because they look at fracture X rays every day. They read bone characteristics from those pictures the way you read joy, fatigue, or worry in the faces of your friends. They know because what they see fits a pattern, not because ordinary X ray is a good way to measure bone strength.

When no characteristic fractures are present, ordinary X rays provide only a rough estimate of bone strength. A bone's density, the tightness of its protein strands and the concentration of the calcium-containing crystals packed into them, is just one determinant of how many X rays pass through and expose the X-ray film. Just as you can identify some people with severe osteoporosis from across the street, doctors can diagnose more advanced cases of decreased bone density from ordinary X rays. A bone must lose about 35 percent of its substance before it appears weak on an ordinary X-ray film. Ordinary X rays are not much help for the milder cases, for people whose bones have not yet become fragile but eventually will without preventive measures, or for measuring changes in bone density.

Doctors have tried to train themselves to make more accurate evaluations of X rays with the naked eye. Some doctors thought that they could count the number of trabeculations (thick strands within bones that can be seen on hip and spinal X rays) and thus estimate bone strength. That technique has not proven to be very helpful, however, and adds little to the general, naked-eye impression of the film.

Researchers have made careful attempts to control the errors that limit the usefulness of ordinary X ray for diagnosing osteoporosis. The skill of the naked eye has been surpassed by caliper measurements of the thickness of bone edges. Doctors also compare X-ray images of bone to aluminum wedges of known density X-rayed at the same time. A more accurate method is radiographic absorptiometry. Two X rays of the same hand are taken with different voltage settings on the two exposures. The films are then analyzed for bone density. Although any doctor who learns the technique can take the X rays, the analysis is usually done at a medical center with specialized equipment. A nonprofit service is available for this test at Miami Valley Hospital, Yellow Springs, Ohio.

Radiographic absorptiometry can gauge bone density with ten times the accuracy of regular X ray. It is precise enough to determine whether bone density is getting better or worse. The technique is a little cumbersome in that films must be sent away for analysis. Even on a nonprofit basis, the combined costs of taking the X rays, mailing them out, and analyzing them amounts to more than one hundred dollars. Measurements of finger bones may not always correlate with the status of other bones. Although you receive minimal X-ray exposure from a single hand X ray, repeated exams may be cause for concern if your hands have had considerable other X-ray exposure.

CAT SCANS Computers are capable of analyzing ordinary X rays that have been passed through the body at multiple angles and producing images from that analysis. The images resemble X-ray pictures except that they are formed in planes, such as cross sections, which would be impossible in any ordinary picture. The technique is called *computerized axial tomography* (CAT), and the image is called a *CAT scan,* or *CT scan.* The CAT scan is like a slice, taken at a particular level, at a particular plane, and, to a certain extent, at a particular thickness chosen by the doctor. The doctor can choose location, direction and thickness of slices, just as you might choose how to slice an apple.

The thickness of the pillars of bone (trabeculae) can be measured on a CAT scan. The doctor can make a similar evaluation by measuring the pores in solid bone. A fairly accurate assessment of bone density and strength results from such measurement.

CAT scans make deep bones, such as those in the spine, accessible to accurate measurement of osteoporosis. The disadvantages are that CAT scans are expensive and time-consuming. The amount of X ray you receive from a CAT scan, while not excessive for one examination, may worry you if you need repeated tests. You get more radiation from a CAT scan than from radiation absorptiometry or photodensitometry.

ISOTOPE TESTS The smallest particle of matter that retains characteristics of familiar materials is called an atom. Atoms are made up of tiny particles called protons, neutrons, and electrons. The common name for a particular atom depends upon its composition. Similar atoms are said to be of the same element. An element may exist in more than one form. To retain its identity as a particular element, each of its atoms must have the same number of protons. The number of neutrons may vary slightly, but atoms with the same number of protons are all called by the same element name, such as carbon, oxygen, or iodine. Atoms with the same number of protons but different numbers of neutrons are called isotopes.

An isotope is given a number indicating the total number of protons and neutrons it contains—for example, iodine 125. Most elements have one or more stable isotopes that do not give off an appreciable amount of radiation. Those stable isotopes are what make up our bodies and most of the world we see around us. Other isotopes of the same elements may be unstable, meaning they give off radiation and undergo relatively rapid changes in composition. Such unstable isotopes that give off radiation are said to be radioactive. For example, iodine 125 is a radioactive isotope of the stable atom iodine 127.

When radioactive forms of stable elements that occur in the body are injected into the body, they are attracted to certain organs, where they mix with their naturally occurring counterparts. Doctors gain information about an organ when they measure the radiation given off by the radioactive isotope that was injected. Although it may sound unappealing to have radioactive materials injected into your body, remember that the doses are very small. Such techniques have been commonly used in hospitals for many years.

The isotope materials most often injected into the body for bone study are phosphates "labeled" with radioactive technetium. The test is called a *bone scan*. Bone scans help to identify unrecognized fractures and patterns of unusual bone activity. Ordinary bone scans help diagnose osteoporosis only in ways similar to ordinary X rays used for that purpose. The quantity of the uptake cannot be measured well enough to help with early diagnosis or reproduced well enough to measure response to treatment.

Total body calcium, a useful gauge of osteoporosis, can be safely and accurately measured by a technique called *neutron activation*. In this process the whole body is bombarded with neutrons—this sounds terrible, but it isn't. The change that the neutrons create in calcium isotopes can be measured and conclusions can be reached about the body's calcium content. At this time, the test is quite expensive and not generally available.

The most practical use of isotopes for prevention and care of osteoporosis, *photon absorptiometry*, does not require their injection into the body. The isotopes are placed in a container that releases the radiation in carefully controlled beams. Photon absorptiometry requires no X-ray machine and no X-ray film. During the most common test, a single beam from a radioactive iodine source is passed across the forearm. There is no pain. The dose is about 1 percent of the radiation obtained from an ordinary forearm X ray.

Single photon absorptiometry, often called *photodensitometry*, is not available everywhere, but many centers that treat osteoporosis now have it. It takes very little time, and the results are immediate. The cost of an examination varies, but it is usually about one hundred dollars.

Photodensitometry measures bone density more accurately than ordinary X ray. Its accuracy is about the same as that of a CAT scan or radiographic absorptiometry. Since there is a wide range of normality for photodensitometry of the forearm, the process is best used to gauge whether your bones are getting better or worse rather than for a diagnosis or prognosis based upon a single examination.

Some researchers criticize photodensitometry for measuring forearm bones, since the condition of those bones may not be the same as that of the spine or hips. Other research studies have shown, however, that findings from forearm photodensitometry do correlate with total body calcium values as determined by neutron bombardment and with density as determined from bone biopsies taken from lumbar vertebrae. Whether forearm photodensitometry measurements are a valid basis for prediction of whether the bones of the spine will fracture is the question in greatest doubt concerning the value of this measurement technique.

Two different beams from radioactive sources of two different isotopes are used to perform what is called *dual photon absorptiometry*. This technique accurately measures bone density in the spine. In 1980 a Swedish study showed that bone density as determined by dual photon absorptiometry was directly related to bone strength measured by compressing the bone between two metal plates. The study was important because it showed that dual photon absorptiometry was valuable and also because it showed that every little increase in bone density increased resistance to fracture. The problems with dual photon absorptiometry are that it is expensive, time-consuming, and not available except in a few large centers.

Compton scatter, which derives its name from the physics principle it utilizes, provides measurements that depend upon the density of the interior mesh of the bone, whereas photon absorptiometry depends more upon the outer shell. Compton scattering occurs when a beam of high-energy photons from a radioactive source passes through a substance; some of the photons collide with electrons in the substance and change direction. The number of photons that change direction is proportional to the number of electrons in the substance and therefore reflects the density of the substance. Compton-scatter values from forearm bones may give better estimates of spine strength than photon absorptiometry values. Research data about Compton scatter, much of it from Israel, look very promising. The technique has not been tested much outside of research centers and is not readily available to most patients.

BIOPSY   The crushing of bones between metal plates, such as in the Swedish study mentioned above, is done only when bones have been removed after death. However, small pieces of bone can be removed from living people with little pain or risk. Doctors can test the bone of such biopsy specimens in ways that cannot be done on bone still present in the living body.

Sometimes doctors ask their patients to "label" a bone before a biopsy. This is done by having the patient take the antibiotic tetracycline for a designated period before the biopsy is performed. The tetracycline will be visible in the bone that was formed while the patient was taking the antibiotic.

Tests on bone biopsy specimens include microscopic analysis, electron microscopic analysis, specialized X rays, and specialized chemical analyses, including a combination chemical and microscopic study called histochemistry. Except for ordinary light microscope analysis, all of these techniques are usually used for research rather than for helping patients with personal decisions about diagnosis and treatment.

Bone biopsy is a good method for studying osteomalacia, which, as you will learn in Chapter 4, is a disease that is much like osteoporosis and may coexist with it. The surgeon usually takes a sample for bone biopsy from the patient's pelvic bone, just below and in back of the bony prominence you can feel with your fingertips when you stand with your hands on your waist. The doctor cores out a piece of bone about one-quarter of an inch in diameter.

Bone quality varies a great deal from one spot in the body to another. That variation makes it difficult to make judgments about osteoporosis from bone biopsies. Even though the bone that is removed can be tested with extreme accuracy, chance variations in the site of removal can make big differences in the results. Unlike tests done on living bone, the test cannot be repeated upon the same piece of bone at a different time; therefore, effects of treatment must be evaluated from bone taken from different sites—a potential source of error.

Under most circumstances, bone biopsy is not a very good way to study ordinary osteoporosis. Obtaining the specimen is expensive and painful, and the techniques of studying the bone are very demanding. In a few centers, efforts to overcome the problems of biopsy are being made, and in selected cases, biopsies have been beneficial to diagnosis and treatment response of idiopathic osteoporosis.

SUMMARY: DIAGNOSIS OF OSTEOPOROSIS

The above discussions may seem to cover a long and complicated array of tests, but you do not have to remember all that information. Many of the tests are seldom used. New uses for the tests and additions to them are always being made, so it is impractical to stay current unless you are doing research on the subject. Just remember that there are such tests. Refer back to the discussion if you need to review specific information.

Most diagnoses of osteoporosis can be made accurately without any tests at all. After reading this chapter, you will be very good at recognizing it yourself. Your doctor, without needing to prescribe any tests, is very good at diagnosing osteoporosis.

There are some tests that are appropriate for people who are uncertain about the diagnosis of osteoporosis or who are going to be given osteoporosis treatments. A standard blood count and blood chemistry profile, including thyroid-function studies, rule out most underlying causes of osteoporosis. X rays should be taken if fractures are suspected.

If you are being treated for osteoporosis or if you think your risk of developing the disease is high, you should be tested at

TABLE 2
Common Tests for Osteoporosis

Test	*Approximate Cost* *
Physician: History and Physical	$ 50.00
Routine Blood Tests	
Complete Blood Count	10.00
Blood Chemistry	20.00
Thyroid Hormone Levels	50.00
Specialized Blood Tests	
Parathyroid Hormone Level	100.00
Vitamin-D Level	100.00
Protein Electrophoresis	25.00
Arthritis Profile	35.00
Estradiol, Serum	50.00
X Rays	
Lumbar Spine (3 views)	50.00
Pelvis	25.00
Hand	25.00
CAT Scan Lumbar Spine	500.00
Radiographic Absorptiometry	100.00
Isotopes	
Bone Scan (technetium)	200.00
Photodensitometry (single)	120.00
Biopsy	
Surgeon's Fee	250.00
Hospital (outpatient surgery)	400.00
Pathologist's Fee (light microscope only)	50.00

*Fees for medical tests are based upon many quality control factors unrelated to material costs; therefore, fees vary greatly among different laboratories and hospitals.

intervals. The results of earlier tests can be compared in a meaningful way to results obtained from the same tests at a later date. Such tests should be safe, convenient, and reasonably inexpensive. Either photodensitometry or radiographic absorptiometry qualifies.

Unfortunately, at the present time not everyone has easy access to photodensitometry or radiographic absorptiometry. With a little effort, though, you can arrange to have one of those tests. Photodensitometers are available in most urban medical communities. If there is no photodensitometer in your area, your doctor or one of his colleagues can arrange radiographic absorptiometry for you. Repeated testing at prescribed intervals, using one of those tests, is not current standard practice, but it should be and soon will be. You should encourage your doctor to provide one of those services.

Accurate assessments of diagnosis and prognosis of osteoporosis are not difficult. The fact that osteoporosis does not often occur as an isolated medical problem has, in the past, made doctors and patients reluctant to tackle those assessments. As you will read in the next chapter, osteoporosis often occurs coincidentally with other medical conditions. Before you assess your risk, involvement, or future regarding osteoporosis, you should understand what conditions may be coincidental to osteoporosis and not really related to it.

2

Health Problems Associated with Osteoporosis

CERTAIN CONDITIONS occur along with osteoporosis so often that it is important to distinguish their effects. We discussed some common physical characteristics of people with osteoporosis in Chapter 1, so that you could better predict your risk of developing osteoporosis. In Chapter 3 we will discuss several diseases that may be direct causes of osteoporosis. This chapter will deal with conditions that may develop at the same time as osteoporosis but are not necessarily related either as coexisting heredity factors or as causes. Some of the conditions we will discuss here are diseases and others, like menopause and the effects of aging, are normal life processes.

MENOPAUSE

The symptoms of menopause are not likely to be confused with those of osteoporosis, but there is good reason for people who are concerned about osteoporosis to pay particular attention to these symptoms. During and after menopause, women lose calcium from their bones and lose bone strength more rapidly.

The number of years of life after menopause correlates very well with bone weakness.

Menopause, also called the climacteric, generally refers to the changes that women undergo as their reproductive organs change in middle life. Although menopause affects the whole body, the organs central to its occurrence are the ovaries. Each month, from early adolescence until middle life, normal ovaries produce a mature ovum and hormones that prepare the body either to support a pregnancy if that ovum is fertilized or to carry on the cycle the following month if it is not. Sometime between the ages of forty and sixty, normal ovaries stop functioning to support reproduction. They produce ova irregularly at first and then not at all. Their hormonal functions change.

Since about twenty-one million women in the United States are currently experiencing some symptoms of menopause, it can hardly be considered an abnormal occurrence. If active ovaries are surgically removed or if they become inactive because of some disease, menopause may occur at an earlier age and, in that respect, be considered abnormal. Men are also said to undergo a menopause, but the term as applied to men is really a metaphor for changes that men undergo in midlife; they are not really the same as those that women experience.

Sometimes the terminology can be confusing. The word "menopause" is used to refer to many different aspects of these changes. Sometimes menopause is used more precisely to mean the date of the last natural menstrual period. Symptoms of hormone changes that were harbingers of the menopause are then referred to as premenopause and all events after the last period as postmenopause. Most often, in common usage, menopause means the few years before and just after the last natural period, the years when women are apt to experience symptoms as a result of changes in the production of reproductive hormones.

Some women experience vaginal bleeding after menopause. The most common cause of this bleeding is prescribed hormones. Any postmenopausal vaginal bleeding not explained by prescribed hormones calls for concern and immediate consultation with a physician.

Every year about 650,000 women have hysterectomies, surgical removal of the uterus. In about 30 percent of these cases, the ovaries are removed at the same time. If the ovaries and uterus are removed, the operation is properly called a hysterectomy and oophorectomy; if the fallopian tubes are also removed, the procedure is called a hysterectomy and salpingo-oophorectomy. That gets to be a lot of syllables, so many times people simply refer to all such operations as hysterectomies.

Unless you know exactly what was removed, you cannot predict the effect it will have regarding osteoporosis and many other factors. Whether you have not yet experienced menopause, are experiencing symptoms of menopause now, or are long past all that, it is important, when making decisions about osteoporosis, that you understand which of these changes your body has undergone or will undergo, and at what ages.

If your uterus has been removed, you will not get pregnant, will not have menstrual periods, and will not have to worry about cancer of the cervix and uterus (provided you did not have any sign of such at the time of the operation). If your ovaries were working normally at the time your uterus was removed and the surgeon left them in, you will probably not have any major hormonal changes as a result of the operation. You will not experience any symptoms of menopause other than cessation of periods. I say "probably" because some women do experience such changes because their ovaries, even though not removed, stop functioning after their hysterectomies.

Whether normal, functioning ovaries should be removed at the time of hysterectomy is controversial. The reason most often given for removing ovaries is to eliminate the risk of cancer. The risk that a woman who has had a hysterectomy will develop ovarian cancer is somewhere between one in one hundred and one in one thousand. Any risk of cancer is cause for concern, but when one considers that one woman in twelve develops breast cancer, and one woman in twenty-five colon cancer, and that those organs are not removed when they are normal, the practice of removing normal ovaries becomes less compelling. Stronger cases can be made for removing nonfunctioning ovaries or ovaries from women who have reason to consider themselves at high risk for cancer. As far as osteoporosis is concerned, however, it is better not to have your ovaries removed, especially if they have years of active function left in them.

If you have a hysterectomy and your ovaries are removed, from that moment your body is postmenopausal. That knowledge helps explain symptoms you may experience, and it is especially important to your plans to protect yourself from the effects of osteoporosis. If you have a hysterectomy and your ovaries are left in, but you then experience other symptoms of menopause, you must consider that your ovaries may have quit functioning and that your risk of osteoporosis has increased from that time.

If you have a hysterectomy, your ovaries are left in, and you experience no symptoms of menopause at that time, it is likely that your ovaries are still working to protect your bones. However, you must realize that your ovaries will one day stop functioning. When that happens, your body will experience menopause, but you will not have the clues of menstrual irregularities and finally cessation of periods that signal menopause to most women. You will need to be especially alert to other symptoms of menopause and, if in doubt, you may need laboratory tests of hormone function.

When ovaries stop functioning in the ways they do during the reproductive years, an array of symptoms may occur. Some of these menopause symptoms are easily explained by hormone changes and are surely related to the menopause; others may only be coincidentally related.

The best-known and most dramatic symptom of menopause is the hot flush, frequently called "hot flash." About 35 percent of women have hot flushes in the premenopausal and postmenopausal years. Nearly 70 percent experience at least some of the effects of hot flushes. A woman having a hot flush behaves exactly as anyone does who is too hot, but the stimulus is internal. The pulse races, the skin flushes red, and perspiration increases. Most women who have hot flushes have them for more than one year, and many women have them for more than five years.

Thinning of the hair, dryness of the skin and vagina, and sagging of the breasts are predictable accompaniments of menopause. Many other symptoms are reported by more than 25 percent of women during the few years before and after the menopause. They include nervousness, tiredness, insomnia, depression, joint pain, muscle pain, headache, backache, memory deficits, and bladder incontinence. Whether these symptoms are physically caused by the hormonal changes of menopause or whether they are just coincidental to women in the menopause age group is controversial. The subject will be discussed at greater length in Chapter 5.

About 20 percent of women lose bone mass very rapidly, much more rapidly than other women, during the years around the time of menopause. About 25 percent of women have dramatic symptoms of menopause, such as severe hot flushes. These two groups are not the same. You cannot predict on the basis of symptoms of the menopause whether or not you are losing bone more rapidly than the average woman of your age. You may be a rapid bone-loser during menopause even if you have little or no trouble with the symptoms of menopause. Regardless of the severity of the symptoms, you lose bone strength more rapidly than you did before and you need extra precautions, then and thereafter, to protect yourself from the complications of osteoporosis.

PREGNANCY AND MOTHERHOOD

Symptoms of osteoporosis seldom occur during pregnancy, since women who are young enough to be pregnant are seldom old enough to experience osteoporosis. Some statistics even show that women who have had children are less likely to show signs of osteoporosis later in life than women who have not borne children. Heredity, hormonal influences, and social factors may explain such statistics.

However, if you consider the nutritional demands of pregnancy, you will find good reasons to be concerned that pregnancy may aggravate osteoporosis. The recommended daily allowance of dietary calcium more than doubles during pregnancy and breast feeding. Since fewer than 33 percent of American women have enough calcium in their regular diets, a woman may have to quadruple her usual calcium intake during pregnancy and for as long as she breast-feeds her baby. If she does not take in that much calcium, her body will maintain a normal calcium level in her blood and provide the necessary calcium for the baby at the expense of her bones.

Hormonal factors encourage replacement of withdrawals from the bone bank during pregnancy and breast feeding; but unless deposits, in the form of a very high calcium diet, are made, the calcium balance in the skeleton will be reduced. If you anticipate pregnancy, you can use this information to help prevent osteoporosis. If you have already had pregnancies during which you have not dramatically increased your calcium intake, you must consider the loss you sustained then as you assess the current status of your bones.

OLD AGE

One out of every nine Americans is over sixty-five. By the year 2020, one in five Americans will be over sixty-five and one in ten will be over seventy-five. Old age was once equated with inability to work, have fun, and otherwise participate in life. However, numerous examples of productive, creative people in their seventies, eighties, and nineties prove that such is not always the case.

The diseases that affect older people are now better understood. It has become increasingly clear that chronic disease, not age, is the reason so many older people cannot function. One of today's most compelling medical challenges is to distinguish the effects of age from those of chronic disease; the challenges of the future are to prevent and to further ameliorate the symptoms of chronic disease.

We once thought that heart disease was an inevitable consequence of aging; we now know that hearts free of coronary artery blockage from arteriosclerosis will function normally in advanced age. We also know that proper diet and exercise and healthful habits can keep coronary arteries open. We once thought that mental confusion and senility were the inevitable results of aging; we now know that people who are free of Alzheimer's disease, arteriosclerosis of the arteries to the brain, and other causes of brain dysfunction can maintain sharp intellectual and creative abilities into very advanced ages.

Social isolation makes depression a common problem among older people, but that is an environmental circumstance that responds to change, and is not a consequence of aging. Depression and loneliness lead to inactivity, which leads to weak bones and other problems common among older people. The problem is the depression, not aging. As you get older, your physical and mental health require that you be around other people.

Loss of function due to poor leg circulation results from disease of the blood vessels, not just age. Many elderly people have perfectly normal circulation in their legs. You can help prevent poor circulation in old age if you eat the right foods and avoid tobacco when you are young. The condition of many people who already have poor circulation in their legs can be improved with medicines or surgery.

All joints slowly stiffen. Most of the various forms of arthritis lead to loss of joint function, which progresses with age. Stiffness, instability, and pain in joints once forced people to severely limit their activities and lose function as they aged. They lost function because they had bad joints, not because they were old. Now, anti-inflammatory medicines, proper exercises, and joint replacement operations keep people active in spite of joint disorders.

We once thought that stooped backs and broken hips and wrists were unavoidable banes of the aged. We now know how to prevent and cure osteoporosis.

Many problems that accompany old age are poorly understood and not easily remediable. Many older people cannot see or hear well. Many chronic diseases, once established, can be only partially controlled. Balance and coordination often diminish with age. Those problems increase the risk of falls and other injuries. However, the presence of those problems does not mean that the effects of osteoporosis should also be present. The complications of osteoporosis are due to a specific treatable and preventable disease, not to old age. If you take care to preserve your bone strength, your bones will resist breakage from minor injury regardless of your age.

ARTHRITIS

Arthritis is a large and complex subject, especially when considered as part of evaluation for risk of osteoporosis. It will be treated fully in Chapter 4.

3

Healthy Bones, Damaged Bones

MOST PEOPLE first learn about bones when they throw out the garbage or feed the dog. Later, they may see fossilized pieces of bone in a museum or bones strung together on wires to make a skeleton for biology class. Few people are introduced to bone as a dynamic, mysterious, adaptable organ the way they are introduced to the heart or the brain. Many people do not think of bone as an organ, much less appreciate how it marvelously adapts form to function and balances a myriad of vital chemical processes.

The shape of your bones determines the shape of your body. Your view of yourself is, in large part, determined by your bones. Your bones are firm, hard, and relatively inflexible, so the shape of your body stays relatively constant. That same firmness provides support and protection for soft tissue organs such as the heart and lungs. The latter are often called "vital organs," but bones are vital organs, too.

Bones are hard because they contain minerals. The rich supply of minerals does not simply lie in the bones to make them hard, like a piece of chalk. Bone is a reservoir of essential minerals for the rest of your body. Bone is the body's major bank for calcium, phosphate, magnesium, sodium, carbonate, and other important ions (the combining forms of atoms or groups of atoms).

In living bone the minerals are not just stored there; they are available because there is an active circulation of blood through the bone and a constant chemical interchange between bone and body fluids. The bank is not just rich in assets; it is constantly open and doing business.

BONE GROWTH

Bones do wonderful things for the body, but the body pays a price. Bone is expensive: much protein and minerals are required to make a bone. The maintenance costs are high too, since bone constantly replaces itself. And the transportation costs are also high, since bone is heavy for the body to carry. Therefore, it is advantageous for the body to make as little bone as needed for necessary functions and for withstanding stress.

Bones are not straight, hollow tubes. All sorts of curves in them provide for body shape, and knobs on them serve as attachments for muscles. For centuries, no one understood how the tiny bones of infants grew into the perfect forms that suit adult life. John Hunter, a famous eighteenth-century bone surgeon, said it seemed that bones had a sort of consciousness—minds of their own that directed their growth.

Such scientific mysteries are often solved in strange ways. The solution to the mystery of bone growth began in 1736, when a London printer invited a young surgeon, John Belchier, to dinner. Belchier noticed a ruddy, red staining in the bones of the roast pig served by his host. Fortunately for science, Belchier was not too polite to inquire about the discolored bones. The printer revealed that he had been feeding bran to his pigs. The bran had been soaked with madder, a plant whose roots and berries serve as sources of red dye. Belchier fed animals madder and then examined their bones. If he stopped giving the animals madder and fed them regular food for a while before they were killed, their bones did not look red from the outside. Cut bones, however, showed a red layer beneath the surface. Belchier reasoned that bones, like trees, grew by depositing new layers around the outside. He had discovered a way to measure that growth.

Although Belchier's early experiments with madder demonstrated how bones grow larger around, they did not explain how bones grow longer or how the central marrow cavity enlarges. A theory that bones grow longer from the middle of their shafts was disproven. Spaced pellets embedded in the shafts of growing bones were found to be no further apart when the bones were reexamined after growth.

John Hunter puzzled about how the knobs and curves of bones remained in appropriate size and location as bones grew. He reasoned that parts of bones must resorb (be absorbed or dissolved) and reform; that as they grow, bones must constantly restore themselves in new forms—a process called "remodeling." He drew those correct conclusions in 1754, almost a century before scientists recognized that living matter was made up of tiny cells and particles that could be studied with microscopes.

In 1853, Scottish surgeon John Goodsir studied bone cells with a microscope. He discovered that a bone grows longer because new bone forms near the ends of the bone. Those growth sites, called "epiphyseal growth plates" (sometimes, imprecisely, "epiphyses"), remain open and active until growth ceases. Long bones do not grow in length after late adolescence; when the epiphyseal plates close, the sites of the growth cells seal themselves and harden.

Goodsir's work did not stop with examination of human bones. Again, human science progressed because inquiring minds of scientists were open to clues from improbable sources. Goodsir and his students examined sponges dredged from the waters of Spitzbergen, Norway. Sponges were easy sources for the study of cells in those early days of microscopy. Goodsir's group not only studied the form of the cells; they also noted the patterns the cells formed in their relationships to one another. The geometric patterns of the sponge cells and spicules, which the cells produce during growth, were in the exact position and size the sponge needed for support. When the scientists rotated a sponge so that waves struck it from a different angle, its growth changed to provide strength where it was needed.

In the late 1800s, Julius Wolff, an orthopedic surgeon in Berlin, observed many details of how human bones undergo changes similar to those that occurred in Goodsir's sponges. Wolff called his conclusions "The Law of Bone Transformation," but the rest of the world has called them "Wolff's Law." Wolff's Law states that bone elements rearrange themselves and grow smaller or larger in response to stress. Not only do bone cells perform these functions, but they do so according to mathematical laws, constructing new supports in form, size, and position that would meet the approval of expert engineers. It seems that John Hunter was right when he said that bone seemed to have a consciousness of its own.

In summary, bones grow in three ways. During childhood, they grow longer by adding new bone near their ends. They grow bigger around by depositing thin layers of bone on their outside surfaces, like a tree. And they constantly tear down and rebuild themselves in order to shape new growth to the adult form and to respond to stress.

The long bones of adults do not grow longer; however, other forms of bone growth continue throughout life. Imagine that you have constructed a building. Once the building is finished, you add no new rooms. You keep the size and general shape of the building the same, although you make some minor changes in the outside surface contours, on the order of shutters or flower boxes. You add a few coats of paint to the outside. You constantly remodel and reinforce the supporting beams and walls.

After many years, a building such as the one described would still be about the same size and shape as it was just after it was completed, even though the supports and the materials that compose it may have undergone considerable change. That is roughly, though not exactly, the situation with bones. What usually happens in bone is that the inside surfaces of the walls are stripped away more than they are replaced. What thickness the walls lose from the inside remodeling is partially replaced by the new paint or siding added to the outside. In old age, therefore, bones are larger around and have larger interior spaces and thinner walls than in young adulthood. The fact that they are larger around becomes important as a safeguard against breakage. A 10 percent increase in diameter compensates for a 30 percent decrease in mass when measuring resistance to certain forces that could cause a bone to break.

BONE STRUCTURE

Although bones may vary in external shape, they have certain similarities in structure. It will help to understand osteoporosis and fractures if you can form an accurate image of the basic structure of bone. Although it is not essential to intelligent self-care, you may find it interesting to learn some of the vocabulary of bone structure.

As we have said, bones are not hollow tubes: they have a dense, hard outer shell and a more lacelike interior. Some bones, like the vertebrae of the spine, have structures similar to a baked biscuit—the compact outer crust is relatively thin and the center is filled with multiple solid strands, loosely woven around small, scattered cavities. In long bones the outer crusts are thicker, the central structures sparser, and the central cavities larger. The ends of long bones are bigger around than their shafts. The bone structure near the bulbous ends of long bones is more biscuit-like. The outer crust of bone is called the *cortex* (plural, "cortices"), the woven beams of the interior are called *trabeculae*, and the cavities are called *marrow spaces*.

Just as in building construction, bones are constructed most efficiently with beams, in this case the trabeculae. The cost, in terms of materials, is much less to build with beams than to build solid structures. The strength, relative to the weight, is much greater with beams. Since the body transports its structure from place to place, the strength-to-weight ratio is very important.

While the overall form of a bone must remain fairly constant, the internal structure can be rearranged to suit changing needs, an adaptability well provided for by trabecular beam construction. The loose weaving is also important to the reservoir function of bone, because it provides surfaces that are easily accessible to body fluids.

A bone's structure must allow it to function as a living, reacting organ constantly remodeling itself and supplying essential elements to the rest of the body. You will understand how bone structure facilitates those functions if you think of the surfaces of bone.

Most people think of bone as having only one surface—the outer surface that one sees when looking at a whole bone. However, if you imagine that you are a calcium ion in solution, circulating through bone, you will visualize three bone surfaces. As you circulate in the blood on the outer surface of the bone, you follow a parallel course through miles of tiny vessels running through a smooth sheet of tissue folded around the bones. This tissue, called the *periosteum,* forms an envelope around the outside surface of a bone. The periosteum is easy to see and peel away from the bone. At most sites it is a bit thicker than the skin of a peach. At intervals, there are vessels that join the circulations of the surrounding muscle and the interior of the bone.

As you circulate in the center of the bone, you face another surface. The inside surface of bone lines all the cavities and trabeculae and the inner layers of the cortex. This inside envelope, called the *endosteum,* is much thinner and more irregular than the periosteum. The endosteum cannot be peeled away in a continuous piece of tissue like the periosteum. The endosteum is marked with irregular pools and crannies; because of this, its total surface is much greater than that of the periosteum.

There is yet one more surface, even more gossamer and discontinuous than the endosteum. As you circulate from either the

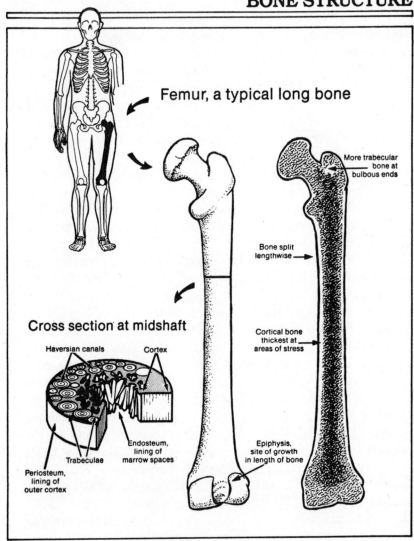

Femur, a typical long bone

More trabecular bone at bulbous ends

Bone split lengthwise →

Cortical bone thickest at areas of stress →

Epiphysis, site of growth in length of bone

Cross section at midshaft

Haversian canals

Cortex

Trabeculae

Endosteum, lining of marrow spaces

Periosteum, lining of outer cortex

endosteum or the periosteum into the dense cortex of the bone, you travel through an intricate system of horizontal and vertical canals. Many of these canals are too small for blood cells, so that only fluids and ions pass through. Their walls are hardened with mineral crystals. This cortical surface, sometimes called the "Haversian surface," is very large because there are so many channels. It is the site of constant, vital activity.

Because of continuous circulation and chemical activity, bone tissue completely replaces itself about every seven years. The overall structure may remain fairly constant, but the tiny protein molecules and mineral crystals that compose it are replaced.

You may compare a living bone to a dynamic city. There is a constant flow of traffic. Some of that traffic brings in supplies, some of it removes materials for use elsewhere. Old buildings are replaced when they are no longer useful. The size, form, and strength of new buildings are determined by need. The following sections describe the construction workers (living cells), the building materials, and the communication systems used to signal the need for demolition or new construction.

BONE CELLS   There are three specialists in the bone construction business.

Bone that is in need of replacement or is no longer useful is removed by *osteoclasts*. Osteoclasts are large cells with more than one nucleus. They accumulate along the bone to be removed and, like so many little Pac Man characters, chew away at the bone surface. Osteoclasts receive some help from circulating blood cells. An active osteoclast can remove twice its own weight in twenty-four hours.

New bone is produced by *osteoblasts*. Osteoblasts are young, energetic cells that not only produce new bone but can also reproduce themselves. After they lay down the basic structure of new bone, the osteoblasts grow up to be *osteocytes*. Osteocytes, which regulate the finishing stages of bone production, are responsible for maintenance. They are tucked away throughout even the most dense parts of bone. They do their solitary job of pumping fluids through tiny channels, regulating mineral contents of bone and fluids, and detecting signs of stress or strain.

MATERIALS   The basic material of bone is the protein *collagen*. Collagen is made of chains of polypeptide molecules wound and braided about one another. Collagen molecules bind together to form long strands called fibrils. As collagen ages, the fibrils form cross-links, so that they coalesce and take some shape. The fibrils are stacked like a wall of bricks with little spaces, or pores. Without the cross-links and the minerals that crystalize in the pores of the fibrils, collagen would be like just so much linguine and not at all like bone.

The main minerals in bone are calcium and phosphate. (Phosphate is a combination of the elements phosphorus and oxygen. Phosphorus is unstable and combines with oxygen so readily that, in nature, it is usually found linked to oxygen.) For a long time, scientists have known that bones are rich in calcium and phosphate. For about fifty years they have thought that most of the calcium and phosphate in bone is in crystals combined as the mineral calcium hydroxyapatite (pronounced like "appetite"). The chemical formula for calcium hydroxyapatite is $Ca_{10}(PO_4)_6(OH)_2$, a piece of information of value only to chemists and the curious. Bone crystals, in fact, contain other combinations of those elements and many elements (such as sodium, potassium, magnesium, strontium, carbon, and chlorine) not part of that formula.

If you set about to make a bone by pouring some calcium and phosphates together, you will be disappointed. If you let the mixture sit for a very long time, you might get a few apatite crystals. Mostly you would just get some chalky calcium phosphate. Even if you got good calcium hydroxyapatite crystals, you would have only a brittle structure with none of the strength of bone.

The strength of bone derives from a healthy combination of strands of collagen and mineral crystals. Separately, neither has much strength; together they form the amazingly strong, adapt-

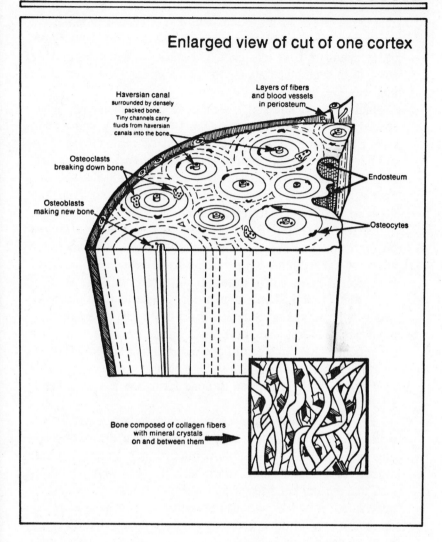

Enlarged view of cut of one cortex

Haversian canal surrounded by densely packed bone. Tiny channels carry fluids from haversian canals into the bone.

Layers of fibers and blood vessels in periosteum

Osteoclasts breaking down bone

Osteoblasts making new bone

Endosteum

Osteocytes

Bone composed of collagen fibers with mineral crystals on and between them able tissue that is healthy bone. This sort of combination is what engineers call a two-phase system. In the twentieth century organic chemists have designed two-phase systems to provide strength in such materials as fiberglass. Bones have been made that way for three hundred million years.

Individual calcium and other ions are incredibly small. When spaced in a latticework of crystals, however, they combine to form a huge surface area. The bone crystals of an average person have a total surface area of about two thousand square miles. Not all of that area is constantly washed by body fluids; some of it is packed away from the erosions of circulating fluid, but the bone cells can get to it if the need dictates.

COMMUNICATION   Bone resorbs—that is, pieces of it are broken down and carted away. Bone reforms—new pieces are added or replace removed parts. But what keeps it all healthy? How does it know where to resorb and where to form? Without some coordination all would be chaos. We know from the beautiful way healthy bones function that it is not chaos. Some communication is local, like workers yelling to each other across a construction site. An area of bone resorption or bone breakdown signals nearby bone cells that some rebuilding is necessary. This marriage of bone resorption to bone formation is called "coupling."

Research scientists have several clues as to how coupling may work. Once we know more about it, the chemical events of coupling may help us understand how osteoporosis is related to hormones, various medicines, and other influences. When the triggers that set off bone resorption and bone formation are better understood, it will be easier to prevent loss of bone health.

At the present time, coupling causes a problem in the treatment of osteoporosis. Some treatments, such as estrogen hormones, decrease bone resorption. That would be more beneficial if it were not for coupling. Because of coupling, when bone resorption decreases, so does bone formation. We need to be able to decrease resorption and increase formation, but coupling frustrates that.

Coupling is the local communication that links resorption to formation. Long-distance communication, like messages from city planners to the local construction crews, may call for either formation or resorption. For long-distance communication to be effective, there must be receivers within the bone, usually called the receptors. The characteristics of those receptors is another subject of research. Understanding receptors is part of the same task as understanding coupling—learning more about the cells and materials of the bone.

We know a little more about the nature of the communications than we do about the receptors. We know that such things as diet, exercise, and hormones communicate about bone resorption and formation to the bones because we can see their effects on the bones of living human beings. We can make similar observations in the laboratory. Bone cells growing in a culture dish will respond to physical forces, electricity, and chemical changes in ways that affect formation and resorption.

WHAT GOES WRONG IN OSTEOPOROSIS?

You can see from what we have covered in this chapter that many different things cause loss of bone. Too many long-distance messages may call for resorption of bone. There may not be enough messages asking the cells to produce bone. The messages can go awry, or the receivers of those messages can be faulty or deficient. Any of the various cells that make, maintain, and resorb bone may work improperly, or there may be too many or not enough of those cells. The coupling communication between building and tearing down may be out of balance. Even if all the communications are effective and the cells are working, if sufficient building materials are not delivered to the site, the job will not be done properly.

We know loss of bone from the cortex, the thick outer layer of bone, is continuous and fairly evenly progressive with age (although, after age fifty, women lose cortical bone about twice as fast as men). Loss of bone from the trabeculae, however, occurs very rapidly just after menopause and then occurs more slowly with advancing age. By age eighty, women have lost about half of their trabecular bone, whereas men have lost only about 15 percent. We know that the bone loss from inactivity is greater in the cortex than in the trabeculae. The different sites of bone loss suggest that all osteoporosis is not the same. Whether cortical or trabecular bone is lost has important implications when we consider where and why bones break. When we understand this better, it may help us to decide how to prevent and treat osteoporosis.

Calcium deficiency, whether because of inadequate diet or inadequate absorption, affects bone in several ways. The body needs to maintain a steady calcium level in its fluids. If the serum calcium level drops, the parathyroid gland broadcasts long-distance signals to the bones to give up some calcium. Whether people with abnormally active parathyroid glands have a distinct form of osteoporosis is controversial. Increased resorption probably causes more trouble than calcium deficiency during formation, although the two aspects of calcium supply are linked and both are important.

Old people absorb less calcium, get less exercise, and have other medical problems that may cause them to lose bone more than they did when they were younger. Those may be sufficient explanations of why men, and women who did not have much increase in bone loss at the time of menopause, develop osteoporosis as they age. Some researchers think that aging osteoblasts simply cannot keep making enough bone and replacing osteocytes fast enough to keep up with normal resorption and death of old osteocytes. Whether the osteoporosis of aging is a distinct process from the osteoporosis that worsens rapidly at menopause is controversial.

Some people, regardless of age, do not seem capable of forming new bone. Even if they do not resorb excessively, their bones weaken because of inadequate formation. Even stimuli to bone formation, such as fluorides, do not lead to increased new bone: about one-fourth of osteoporotic people treated with fluorides do not increase bone formation. Maybe they have a distinct type of osteoporosis.

Previously I noted that you need not worry about the different types of osteoporosis unless you have one of the recognized external causes, such as those discussed in Chapter 2. That is true because we don't know enough to make specific treatment recommendations based upon types of idiopathic osteoporosis. We know that the combination of things we recommend in this book helps almost everyone with osteoporosis.

If we knew exactly what caused an individual's osteoporosis, we could make more exact recommendations as to how much treatment is necessary for that individual. Although we have not reached that point yet, we know much more than we used to know. If you follow the recommendations in this book, you may fuss over certain aspects of osteoporosis more than you would need to if we could tell more precisely where and how great your risks are; nevertheless, if you follow the recommendations, you will make things better for yourself.

WHAT MAKES BONES BREAK?

Bone, like any material, breaks when applied stress exceeds the bone's strength to hold itself together. Of course, different sorts of stresses come to bear upon bones, but the bones do get some external support, primarily from muscles. A bone may break in different ways, ways that are more understandable after you have learned the facts in this chapter. Some bones break all of a sudden, and some break bit by bit.

If you apply stress to an obviously bendable structure, like a coat hanger wire, you will see it bend. What you don't see is that as it bends, an electrical current is produced; the outside, convex side of the bent wire has a charge opposite to that of the inside, concave side. The current not only occurs all along the wire as you see it, but also along each of the little metal crystals of which the wire is composed. The phenomenon of electricity produced as the result of bent crystals is called the "piezoelectric effect."

When stress is applied to bones, they bend. Unlike coat hanger wires, they don't bend enough for you to see. Their behavior is closer to that of a heavy broomstick. If a broomstick is long enough, if a great deal of stress is applied, and if you watch closely, you can barely see it bend. You can reason from that barely visible bend that less force on a shorter stick still creates some bend—under those circumstances, the bend is too small to see.

The bend that occurs to a bone under stress is even less visible than that of a broomstick, because adult bones are more rigid than broomsticks. Whether it is visible or not, bones nonetheless do bend. For the whole bone to bend, the individual trabeculae and cortices must bend. On an even smaller level, bone collagen and bone mineral crystals bend. Since bones are laden with crystals, the piezoelectric effect occurs in bones when the bones bend. I mentioned before that some of the messages sent to bone-producing cells may be electrical messages: the piezoelectric effect is a source of those messages.

If a great deal of stress is applied and rapidly creates a bending force that exceeds the strength of the bone, the whole bone may suddenly break completely through. If the force is very great and very rapid, the bone may almost explode; it may break into more than two pieces, like a shattered glass. On the other hand, if stress is applied slowly and is just enough to bend some parts of the bone beyond their breaking point, cracks may form only in certain parts of the bone and the bone may not break in two. The cracks may be so small that they cannot be seen either by looking directly at the bone or by looking at an X ray of it.

When tiny, invisible cracks form, normal bone responds with a repair process. The cracks are sealed and the weakened areas are shored up by some extra bone, perhaps in response to messages from the piezoelectric effect. If the cracks form too fast or are too large, if the message to form new bone is misdirected or not received properly, or if the repair process is too slow or too weak, the whole bone becomes weak and may collapse or break through.

The final event preceding the breaking of the bone may be a very minor stress, even just a change of posture. Major fractures in bones weakened by osteoporosis occur when stresses exceed the strength of the bones, but that strength may have gradually diminished over many years and for the many reasons discussed throughout this book.

4

Health Problems That Cause Osteoporosis

CHAPTERS 1 AND 2 described the personal traits of people who develop osteoporosis and how osteoporosis relates to life changes. Those characteristics and events apply to the common form of osteoporosis, the idiopathic osteoporosis that is not caused by some other known problem.

Many diseases can cause osteoporosis; however, the combined total of all people with such known causes of osteoporosis makes up only a small minority of the total osteoporosis population. The percentage of osteoporosis patients with some known cause varies in different geographic areas, but is probably about 15 percent overall.

This chapter briefly considers several of the many health problems that can cause osteoporosis. The topics will have special meaning to you if you know that you have had one of these problems. Concern about some underlying cause is also greater if you have osteoporosis and the previously described personal characteristics of idiopathic osteoporosis don't seem to apply to you. If you do not fit the profile of a person who is likely to get osteoporosis and you have been told that you have osteoporosis, then you have more reason to look into the possibility that some of the causes described in this chapter might apply to you.

Keep in mind, too, that osteoporosis is a relative diagnosis. Osteoporosis may not be absolutely present or absent as a light is either on or off. Instead, there is a full spectrum of bone strengths. The underlying causes described here may be the sole causes of osteoporosis, responsible for whatever weakness is present, or they may be minor contributors. Bone that has been partially weakened by the usual mechanisms of idiopathic osteoporosis may be further weakened by mild or brief occurrences of one of the problems described in this chapter.

PERSONAL HEALTH HABITS

Life-style obviously encompasses most of the things we will discuss in this book. Diet, physical vigor, psychological vigor, and reliance on medication are among the personal habits that will be discussed in more detail in other sections. Diet and physical activity are mentioned briefly in this chapter because a discussion of underlying causes of osteoporosis would be incomplete without them. Diet and underexercise are more important as contributors to idiopathic osteoporosis than as solitary causes. Perhaps smoking and alcohol abuse would logically fit into the discussion of drugs as causes of osteoporosis, but most people who smoke or drink alcohol regularly think of those activities more as personal habits than as drug abuse.

SMOKING Smokers get tired of hearing all the terrible things smoking does to their health. Unfortunately, I cannot spare them more of the same regarding osteoporosis. Complicated symptomatic osteoporosis is much more common among smokers than among nonsmokers. The picture of the thin, fair-skinned lady who is stooped from spinal fractures or limping from a broken hip is too often completed by a cigarette between her fingers. We do not know exactly why osteoporosis is worse in smokers, but we do know some things that may be related. Women who smoke experience menopause on the average of five years earlier than women who do not. Smokers do not have good lung function, and they often suffer chronic cough. Shortness of breath makes it harder to exercise. Coughing may cause loss of bladder control during exercise, placing yet another obstacle in the way of enjoying physically vigorous activities. People with chronic lung insufficiency tend to have a little more acid in their blood— a state known as respiratory acidosis. Slight acidity of the blood may increase the mobilization of calcium and other minerals from bone. Nicotine and tobacco resin residues may increase the loss of calcium through the urine.

Smoking interferes with normal circulation, a fact proven by the increased incidence of coronary artery disease, strokes, aneurysms of the major arteries, and gangrene of the feet and legs among smokers. Although it has not been proven that smoking interferes with circulation to the bones, this is a reasonable assumption. It is also reasonable to assume that if bones do not have good circulation they cannot undergo the remodeling and repair processes necessary to maintain strength.

ALCOHOL   We know that alcoholics and people who regularly drink alcohol have worse problems with osteoporosis than nondrinkers. How much is too much? We do not know. For many people, one drink is too much because they cannot stop; for those who can drink moderately, we are not sure about the effect of alcohol on their bones.

We aren't certain why heavy drinkers develop osteoporosis, although we are sure that they do. Alcoholism is probably the most common cause of osteoporosis in men under sixty. Many older women who drink regularly aggravate their idiopathic osteoporosis by their drinking habits.

Alcohol in the intestines decreases absorption of calcium, a problem that is further aggravated by the taking of antacids. Since alcohol irritates the stomach, drinkers tend to take more antacids. As we will discuss later in this chapter, some antacids interfere with calcium absorption. Alcohol also poisons the liver. Normal liver function is necessary to convert vitamin D to its active form. Without active vitamin D, calcium absorption is impaired. Many alcoholics develop physical traits similar to those of people who take cortisone regularly or who have overactive adrenal glands. Osteoporosis is a common characteristic of those people. Finally, the psychological and social impairment of excessive alcohol makes it unlikely that heavy drinkers get the nutrition and exercise they need to maintain healthy bones.

DIET Starvation, anorexia nervosa, and other causes of extreme nutritional deficiency are, by themselves, causes of osteoporosis. More often, inadequate diet is just a contributing factor to idiopathic osteoporosis or osteoporosis with some known cause. Dietary causes and remedies for osteoporosis are discussed in Chapter 6.

DISUSE People who have been bedridden for prolonged periods, those who are paralyzed, and astronauts who experience periods of weightlessness can become osteoporotic solely because of loss of muscle action and weight-bearing stress. Localized forms of osteoporosis occur in bones that have been protected from stress by surgical devices. More often, relatively inadequate exercise simply contributes to osteoporosis, a problem discussed in detail in Chapter 11.

EXCESSIVE STRESS Extreme stress, even if self-inflicted, may cause osteoporosis. There have been recent, well-publicized instances of young women who, while undergoing extreme training regimens for distance running, stopped having menstrual periods and were found to be osteoporotic. Their periods and bones returned to normal when they modified their training programs.

STOMACH, BOWEL, AND LIVER DISEASE

Diseases that interfere with absorption of nutrients from the intestines can cause osteoporosis, or the closely related problem of osteomalacia.

Some people are born unable to absorb fat and, therefore, fat-soluble vitamin D. Others have inborn errors of vitamin-D metabolism in the bowel, liver, or kidneys. Without normal vitamin-D metabolism, a person cannot absorb calcium normally and the bones suffer. Many people are simply intolerant of milk, and are therefore deprived of the richest common source of calcium.

Pancreatitis or other acquired disease of the pancreas, surgical removal of part or all of the stomach, and chronic intestinal diseases all may cause osteoporosis. Common stomach or duodenal ulcers may indirectly cause osteoporosis, because people with ulcers must take antacids, some of which interfere with calcium absorption.

MEDICINES

Drugs may be direct and principal causes of weak bones; more often, drugs aggravate an existing problem with osteoporosis. In the United States people over sixty-five take 25 percent of the drugs, so the age group at risk for complications of osteoporosis is also at risk for aggravating their bone problems by taking certain medicines. Medicines may also deplete bone strength when taken early in life.

ANTACIDS Antacids containing aluminum interfere with calcium metabolism. Not all antacids contain aluminum, but many of the common ones—ALternaGEL, Aludrox, Amphojel, Basaljel, Camalox, Creamalin, Delcid, Di-gel, Estomul, Gaviscon, Gelusil, Kolantyl, Maalox, Mylanta, Riopan, Rolaids, Silain-Gel, and Simeco—do. Aluminum binds phosphate in the bowel. More calcium is lost in the stool when aluminum is present, but that is not the only problem. When the body is deprived of phosphate in the diet, phosphorus is mobilized from the bones and excreted in the urine along with increased urine calcium. The average American spends one hundred ten dollars per year on antacids. That is a great deal of calcium down the drain.

Several antacids—for example, Alka-Seltzer, Alka-2, Alkets, Bisodol, Citrocarbonate, Lo-Sal, Mylicon, Titralac, and Tums —do not contain aluminum. Medicines that control ulcer symptoms by other mechanisms (such as Tagamet and Zantac) do not threaten bones the way antacids containing aluminum do. Calcium carbonate antacids (such as Titralac and Tums) are calcium supplements that may be beneficial to bones.

SEIZURE MEDICINE Many people take diphenylhydantoin (Dilantin) and/or phenobarbital (also primidone and phensoximide) to control seizures. It may be necessary to take such drugs for a long time, perhaps for life. Those drugs may interfere with vitamin-D metabolism in the liver, decrease calcium absorption, and weaken bones. If you need to take any of those drugs, you should be especially mindful of your bone health. You may need calcium and vitamin-D supplements.

ANTIBIOTICS Most antibiotics probably do not interfere with bone metabolism. People usually take antibiotics for such short periods of time that any effect on bone health is minor. However, tetracycline is one antibiotic sometimes prescribed for months or years—for example, to control acne. Those who take it have more calcium in their urine while they are using it. Tetracycline binds to new bone. If you look at bone through a microscope, you can see the effects of tetracycline. Tetracycline also can stain growing teeth. No definite harm to bone from tetracycline has been proven.

Isoniazid is an antibiotic often given over a period of many months to treat tuberculosis. Increased amounts of calcium appear in the urine of people who are taking isoniazid.

DIURETICS Drugs that increase urine volume are called diuretics. They are used to treat high blood pressure, heart failure, and many other conditions. There are many different diuretics, and the chemical reactions by which they work vary greatly.

One diuretic, furosemide (Lasix), increases calcium loss in the urine. It is effective enough to be used in the treatment of people whose calcium levels have become too high. When taken for a long time by people with normal calcium, there is concern that the calcium loss could weaken bones.

Among the most commonly prescribed diuretics are a group of drugs called thiazides (Diuril, Enduron, Esidrix, HTZ, Hydrodiuril, Hygroton, and Zaroxolyn are some examples). Thiazide diuretics decrease calcium loss from the urine. Some physicians have even recommended thiazides as treatment for osteoporosis, an idea that has not been generally accepted. When osteoporosis is a worry and there is a choice of diuretics, there may be some advantage to the thiazides. Thiazide diuretics are especially helpful for patients who try to maintain a healthy calcium intake in spite of a history of urinary tract stones.

VITAMINS AND MINERALS   Details about vitamin and mineral deficiencies are included in Chapters 6 and 7. The instances in which excess vitamins or minerals may cause osteoporosis are rare.

An excess of vitamin A (more than five thousand units per day) may cause bone loss. Excesses of the fat-soluble vitamins A and D can be very dangerous. One of the effects of excess of either of them may be osteoporosis.

A vitamin-A derivative, isotretinoin (Accutane), is a popular and effective treatment for acne. The course of treatment is relatively short, and in recommended doses there is no apparent problem with bone loss. There have been findings of increased calcium mobilization. Fear of bone loss is not sufficient reason for those who need Accutane to avoid it, but those people should at least make a special effort to maintain good bone health habits.

As discussed in Chapter 6, fluoride may be an effective osteoporosis treatment for some people. However, very high doses, inappropriate timing of fluoride treatment, and perhaps the atypical responses of some people have occasionally resulted in the opposite effects—weak or brittle bone.

PAIN MEDICINES AND TRANQUILIZERS   Most pain medicines and tranquilizers probably have no important direct effects on bone. They have the important and harmful secondary effects of decreasing energy, undermining will, and interfering with the pursuit of healthful dietary and exercise practices. For bone health and many other reasons, such drugs should be taken only under the careful management of a physician.

CORTISONE Of all the drugs that cause osteoporosis, the cortisone drugs (also called steroids) are the worst. Occasional injections of cortisone-like drugs into areas of bursitis or short-term (a week or two) cortisone pills for acute conditions seem to do little or no harm to bones. However, people who take steroids over a long period of time frequently develop a particularly severe form of osteoporosis. Spine and rib fractures are especially common to steroid-induced osteoporosis.

Cortisone is a common general term for a group of drugs whose effects are similar to those produced by the hormones of the adrenal cortex, a subject explained in more detail in Chapter 5. Oral forms of cortisone-like drugs (for example, Aristocort, Celestone, Cortef, Cortisone acetate, Decadron, Deltasone, Hydrocortisone, Medrol, Prednisolone, and Prednisone) may be necessary to control such diseases as asthma, lupus and other collagen diseases, and severe rheumatoid arthritis.

High doses of steroids, taken over a long time, increase bone loss and decrease bone formation—in other words, they destroy bone coming and going. They also may cause ulcers, leading to more trouble from antacids. Steroids may cause depression and consequently decrease the likelihood of exercise.

ARTHRITIS

The meaning of the term "arthritis" is already confusing enough. All sorts of conditions are called arthritis, even by medical people. Many times people use the word to refer to any sort of ache or pain in or around a joint. Even when the use is narrowed to refer to diseases that produce abnormalities in joints, it can refer to many different conditions. Rheumatology is a medical specialty that has grown because it is so difficult for doctors to distinguish among the many different forms of arthritis. Unfortunately, when we talk about osteoporosis and arthritis, the subject does not become any simpler, because different forms of arthritis affect osteoporosis in different ways.

The aches and pains of aging are often called arthritis. That is an improper use of the word in the absence of specific abnormal changes in the joints, but we are stuck with it because it is so common that advertising for medicines and even physicians' explanations to patients perpetuate that usage. Joints stiffen with age partly because of normal changes in the tissues of the joints and partly because people exercise less as they age. Stiffness limits joint motion and produces pain with movement, but that is not a joint disease. Stiffness is related to osteoporosis in two ways: both occur in older people and both are aggravated by inactivity.

Injury to a joint, such as a broken bone that extends into the joint, may leave the joint stiff, swollen, or painful. Such a condition is often called arthritis. It is best to distinguish arthritis occurring in a joint after injury as post-traumatic arthritis. That type of arthritis is not a disease and does not result in arthritis in other joints. Post-traumatic arthritis is not associated with osteoporosis unless the severity of the joint disorder limits physical activity enough to weaken bone.

The aches and pains of aging and the effects of injury are most often confused with the most common type of arthritis, osteoarthritis. Osteoarthritis usually worsens slowly with age and is often so mild that changes in the joints are not detectable for years. Osteoarthritis results in thickening of the bone just under the joint surface and around the edges of the joint. Many people can see the effects of their osteoarthritis in the knobby enlargements around the joints at the ends of their fingers. The most disabling sites of osteoarthritis, however, are usually the hip and knee joints.

As painful and disabling as osteoarthritis may be, the good news is that people with osteoarthritis seldom develop severe osteoporosis. People with severe osteoarthritis look different in several respects from those with severe osteoporosis. People with osteoarthritis tend to be bigger, more heavily muscled, and fatter than people with osteoporosis. Although all people who do not take special precautions lose calcium from their bones, those with osteoarthritis lose calcium at a rate only one-third as fast as those with osteoporosis.

People with osteoporosis and people with osteoarthritis constitute large percentages of visitors to the offices of orthopedic surgeons. The orthopedic surgeons notice that the two groups are quite distinct. People with hips severely diseased by osteoarthritis seldom break those hips. When operations are done to replace diseased joints, the difference between cutting through and shaping a bone diseased by osteoarthritis and one affected by osteoporosis is remarkable. Osteoarthritic bone is hard and thick; osteoporotic bone may be like eggshell, with no inner support.

Even though people with osteoarthritis seem to constitute a different group, probably on the basis of heredity, from those with osteoporosis, they still must be concerned about developing osteoporosis. Although osteoarthritic people lose bone less rapidly, they still lose bone unless they make special efforts to prevent loss. Their risk of complications from osteoporosis increases substantially if osteoarthritis limits their physical activities. Lack of exercise, and particularly bed rest, are prime causes of osteoporosis. People with osteoarthritis must stay active if they are to keep their bones strong. Fortunately, modern medicine and joint surgery make it possible for most people to remain quite active in spite of severe osteoarthritis.

Rheumatoid arthritis is very different from osteoarthritis. The two are sometimes confused because they are both common diseases, both are often called arthritis, and both can cripple joints. Many people with rheumatoid arthritis have a rapid progression of joint abnormalities, and so the disease is sometimes called "crippling arthritis," although any true arthritis can be crippling.

Rheumatoid arthritis is a specific, fairly common disease that can be recognized by most physicians. It is usually diagnosed by blood tests. Doubtful cases can usually be diagnosed by a rheumatologist. Some people with joint pain claim they have rheumatoid arthritis, meaning they have severe joint pain. No one should consider himself to have rheumatoid arthritis unless that specific diagnosis has been made by a physician.

The diagnosis of rheumatoid arthritis has special implications regarding osteoporosis. Osteoporosis tends to be worse in people with rheumatoid arthritis. People with rheumatoid arthritis break their hips and other bones more frequently than other people. The total body calcium content of people with rheumatoid arthritis is, on the average, almost 10 percent less than that of other people.

There are several reasons why rheumatoid arthritis may make osteoporosis worse. Rheumatoid arthritis may be very painful, resulting in decreased physical activity. Also, although it is a generalized disease that affects joints dramatically, it also results in muscle wasting, anemia, and general loss of vigor. The appetites of people with rheumatoid arthritis may be poor and their diets inadequate. Since they often take medicines that irritate the stomach, they also take antacids, which may interfere with calcium absorption. Much worse, some people with rheumatoid arthritis have to take cortisone-like drugs that aggravate calcium loss and bone weakness.

There are many other, less common types of arthritis. Most of the relatively uncommon, specific types either occur in people who are more apt to have osteoporosis or cause changes that tend to make osteoporosis worse. Of all the arthritic diseases, only osteoarthritis is associated with decreased risk of osteoporosis. People with osteoarthritis, like those with the joint pains of aging and post-traumatic arthritis, need not fear a direct link of their joint disorder with osteoporosis but must take care to maintain physical activity levels that preserve bone health. People with all other forms of arthritis have reason to consider themselves at increased risk of complications from osteoporosis.

HORMONES

It is especially important for people who are worried about osteoporosis to understand some things about hormones. The definition of hormones and details of the important relationship between various hormones and osteoporosis are provided in Chapter 5. For now, I will simply provide brief descriptions of some diseases related to hormonal disorders.

DIABETES   The best-known hormone disorder is diabetes, a disease in which there is a deficiency of the hormone insulin. People with severe diabetes must take insulin shots daily. In the first six years after diabetes has become severe enough to require insulin injections, there is an increased loss of bone, leading to osteoporosis. After the first six years, the rate of bone loss by insulin-dependent diabetics returns to about the same as that for nondiabetics. However, if the diabetes worsens so that the insulin dose must be increased, there will again be a period of increased rate of bone loss. The result is that the bone mass of the average diabetic person is about 10 percent less than that of nondiabetics of the same age and the risk of complications from osteoporosis is, accordingly, increased for insulin-dependent diabetics.

The relationship of diabetes to osteoporosis has been recognized since 1948. The reasons for the correlation, however, are unknown. Since both problems tend to be hereditary, there may be a genetic link. There could be a relationship between injectable insulin and osteoporosis. Impaired circulation in small blood vessels is a problem for many diabetics and could also contribute to osteoporosis.

THYROID DYSFUNCTION   Hormones from the thyroid gland

regulate the speed of body functions. Underactive thyroid glands cause slow reactions, weak muscles, depression, apathy, intolerance of cold, baggy eyes, dry skin, and deafness—all symptoms often written off as effects of old age. Approximately 3 percent of people over sixty (women more than men) have underactive thyroids. Osteoporosis becomes a problem for them only when they are treated for hypothyroidism, since treatment with thyroid medicines relieves the low-thyroid symptoms but may aggravate the osteoporosis.

An overactive thyroid gland causes speeded-up body reactions, increased pulse rate, high blood pressure, shakiness, nervousness, weight loss, and sometimes bulging of the eyes. An overactive thyroid also causes osteoporosis. Almost 1 percent of women and about 0.1 percent of men over sixty have overactive thyroids. However, elderly people with overactive thyroids often have symptoms that are very different from the ones just described. Irregular heartbeat, heart failure, and enlarged heart occur more often than rapid pulse with high blood pressure. Overactive reflexes and bulging eyes, common in hyperthyroid young people, occur in only 25 percent of older people with overactive thyroids. Older people with overactive thyroids often experience fatigue, depression, and muscle weakness.

Thyroid disorders, which can be discovered by blood tests, can be successfully treated. Since overactive thyroids cause osteoporosis and osteoporosis can result from treatment for an underactive thyroid, people with thyroid disorders must take special care to provide for the health of their bones.

CUSHING'S SYNDROME   Harvey Cushing, an American surgeon generally considered the father of modern neurosurgery, was the first to describe patients whose overactive pituitary glands stimulated their adrenals to produce too much cortisone. Overactive adrenals for any reason can produce Cushing's syndrome, and so can too much cortisone-like medication.

People with Cushing's syndrome have high levels of blood sugar, high blood pressure, fat accumulation in the abdomen, a puffy-looking, moon-faced appearance, muscle weakness, easy bruising, light-colored stretch mark–like streaks on the skin, a "buffalo hump" between the upper shoulder blades, and osteoporosis. The buffalo hump is produced by a fat pad between the shoulders and often because the spine is bent forward by deformity caused by the osteoporosis.

PARATHYROID GLAND ABNORMALITIES   The tiny parathyroid glands in the neck help regulate body calcium. An overactive parathyroid causes osteoporosis. The diagnosis can be made from tests of calcium, phosphorus, and parathyroid hormone levels in the blood. Treatment of the parathyroid abnormalities controls, and often improves, osteoporosis.

SEX HORMONES   The relationship of sex hormones produced by the pituitary gland, adrenals, ovaries, and testes to osteoporosis are discussed in Chapter 5.

CANCER

Many cancers spread to bone. Bone cancers usually weaken specific areas in the bones. Cancer seldom produces generalized osteoporosis throughout the bones; the exception is multiple myeloma, a cancer of the bone marrow that causes generalized bone weakening that may resemble ordinary osteoporosis. Multiple myeloma is a rare disease, and only a tiny fraction of people with osteoporosis have multiple myeloma. X rays of people with multiple myeloma, while sometimes similar to those of people with idiopathic osteoporosis, are usually distinctive enough that physicians suspect myeloma on the basis of the X rays. Results of blood and urine protein tests are usually abnormal, and anemia is often present; a bone marrow examination usually confirms the diagnosis. Therefore, it is quite unusual for people to think they have osteoporosis and be unaware of the presence of multiple myeloma.

If you have osteoporosis with some unusual features and you are worried about cancer, openly discuss your fears with your doctor. Too many people go through their lives worrying about cancer and yet are reluctant to confess their fears to their doctors. Cancer is a very uncommon cause of osteoporosis, so if you are worried it is likely your doctor can reassure you. If tests are necessary, the usual tests are not especially involved, dangerous, painful, or expensive.

HYPERTENSION

The relationships between high blood pressure and osteoporosis are not yet fully understood. A 1981 study from Portland, Oregon, showed that women with osteoporosis had more than double the incidence of high blood pressure compared with women without osteoporosis. Chronic illnesses, because they are associated with decreased exercise and increased need for medications, may contribute indirectly to osteoporosis. In the case of hypertension, however, some data suggest a more complex interrelationship.

We know that calcium deficiency contributes to osteoporosis, and there is some evidence that calcium deficiency may cause high blood pressure. A 1976 study of New Guinean people with low blood pressure showed that the hard water they drank was calcium rich. A 1971–1974 National Center for Health Statistics survey of Americans with high blood pressure showed that the most distinctive nutritional factor was that people with high blood pressure had less calcium in their diets than people with normal blood pressure. Another study, reported in the March 4, 1983, *Journal of the American Medical Association,* showed that increased calcium in the diets of a small group of healthy young adults resulted in a decrease in their blood pressure. Several studies on experimental animals have shown that calcium-poor diets cause blood pressure to go up and calcium-rich diets cause it to come down. Although these and other studies are suggestive, more research is necessary before we can say that calcium deficiency causes hypertension and that calcium deficiency is the link between hypertension and osteoporosis.

OTHER CAUSES OF WEAK BONES

INBORN WEAKNESS   There are several inborn disorders that result in weak bones. They are all rather rare and of concern only to people who develop unusual bone weakness at an early age.

Inborn fragility of the bones, called osteogenesis imperfecta, is often severe and crippling from early life. A mild form, called osteogenesis imperfecta tarda, may result in relatively weak bones throughout life. It does not tend to progress and, in fact, seems to improve as the bones mature. Once mature, however, the bones are subject to the same tendency to become weaker with age as normal bones. Unexplained bone fragility from an early age and a family history of the disease usually identify this rare problem. Some common forms of osteoporosis may be types of osteogenesis imperfecta that manifest themselves late in life—an interesting hypothesis for research but not yet proven or of practical value.

A few other rare diseases—such as Marfan's syndrome, Turner's syndrome, and Gaucher's disease—also cause weak bones. Those diseases are mentioned here only for people who have had such diagnoses made in themselves or their families. Otherwise, you should not worry about them as causes of ordinary osteoporosis in you or your loved ones.

OSTEOMALACIA   Osteoporosis bones are weak because their support structures are too small, like a building constructed without enough large posts and beams to make it strong. If the posts and beams are numerous enough and large enough, but are made of inferior material, the building will be weak for a different reason. Bones whose beams are big enough but are made from inferior materials are said to be affected by osteomalacia.

Osteomalacia occurs when bone forms without enough minerals, especially calcium. If the deficiency occurs in a growing child, the problem is called *rickets* and is a bit different because the bones grow into abnormal shapes. Any adult who is severely calcium deficient for long enough will get osteomalacia. Unlike osteoporosis, osteomalacia occurs in anyone with severe calcium deficiency, not according to the risk criteria for osteoporosis that were discussed in Chapter 1.

Few people have diets so deficient in calcium that they will develop osteomalacia. Milder, long-term calcium deficiency is one of the contributory causes of osteoporosis. Calcium deficiency severe enough to cause osteomalacia is usually due to vitamin-D deficiency, since vitamin D in the diet is necessary for calcium absorption. A vitamin-D deficiency may be caused by inherited errors in the metabolism of vitamin D, inadequate dietary intake of vitamin D, or too little exposure to sunlight. Sunlight causes skin to produce vitamin D from cholesterol. Kidney, liver, stomach, and intestinal diseases and certain medicines all may interfere with the absorption and normal function of vitamin D.

Osteomalacia, in its pure form, differs from osteoporosis in some important respects. Persistent bone pain and tenderness in multiple areas and muscle weakness are more characteristic of osteomalacia, whereas sudden episodes of well-localized pain explained by fractures are more typical of osteoporosis. Osteomalacia causes rib fractures more often than osteoporosis. Microscopic examination of bone samples from people with osteomalacia shows normal sizes and numbers of beams of bone, but too little calcium in those beams. Similar examination of samples from people with osteoporosis shows fewer and smaller beams than normal. People with osteomalacia improve rapidly when they are treated with the appropriate type and dose of vitamin D, but vitamin D does relatively little good for typical osteoporosis.

All that seems fairly clear, but many people have problems

that are not so easily defined. Many people with severe osteoporosis have some osteomalacia as well. Not only are the structures of their bones too few and too small, but they are also calcium deficient. Some degree of osteomalacia is more common among people who drink no vitamin D–fortified milk and get little sunshine. Reports of patients from New York and England suggest that over 10 percent of women with hip fractures have significant osteomalacia.

There is no practical way to detect minor degrees of osteomalacia. The diseases and drugs that increase the likelihood of severe osteomalacia have already been discussed. If those factors apply to you or you have a vitamin D–deficient diet and little exposure to sunlight, you need to discuss the possibility of osteomalacia with your doctor; you may need vitamin-D supplements.

If you do not have diseases or take drugs that would cause osteomalacia, you should take simple precautions to avoid any contribution osteomalacia might make to bone weakness—that means adequate intake of calcium, vitamin D, and a little sunshine. If you cannot get enough vitamin D in your diet, take a supplement, but don't take large doses. Vitamin D can be very dangerous in large doses. If you need treatment for osteomalacia with large doses of vitamin D, take them under the careful supervision of a physician—do not trust such treatment to self-care methods or the advice of health food dealers.

5

Hormones and Osteoporosis

OSTEOPOROSIS may be prevented and, in some cases, treated by taking medicines similar to the natural substances that regulate body functions. Under normal circumstances, these substances, called hormones, circulate in the bloodstream in small and well-defined amounts. Many of the diseases that cause osteoporosis are caused by abnormal hormone function. The common type of osteoporosis, which has no known relationship to other specific diseases, is at least partly related to hormone deficiency.

The study of hormones can be complicated, but you need not be a scientist to understand some of the basic principles. You don't even have to understand all the principles to learn about the effects of hormone treatment. However, the subject is more interesting and your understanding is more complete if you learn how the treatment possibilities relate to normal hormone function. In the first part of this chapter we will consider some of the background information; in the last part we will consider the treatment implications. Don't be put off if the first part is hard to understand when you first read it: it gets simpler as it goes on.

Hormones control four types of body functions. They maintain a steady background, or milieu, for the chemical reactions of the body; they control emergency responses to such stimuli as injury, illness, and psychological upset; they regulate normal growth and development; and they control the specialized functions of sex and reproduction. The last topic will be our concern in this chapter.

Hormones, which have many different chemical compositions, are produced by the endocrine glands, scattered throughout the body. Hormones travel from the endocrine glands through the bloodstream to the sites where hormone action takes place. The study of hormones is called endocrinology. The word "hormone" is derived from a Greek word for stirring up and setting into motion. The term was first applied to biology in 1904, ten years after the first hormone to be isolated, adrenaline, was identified.

Endocrine glands are not necessarily located near the sites where their hormones act. A small gland in one part of the body may have widespread effects because its hormone is carried through the bloodstream. However, there is a tendency for the glands to be located near the sites where they are most active. The ovaries and testes, for example, are near the reproductive organs, yet their hormones have far-reaching effects on all the bones of the body.

Few body functions are influenced by only one hormone; most body functions are controlled by many. Each hormone has several effects, rather than only one. Bone, the focus of our interest in this subject, is a good example. Many different hormones affect bone, but those hormones, for the most part, are better known for their actions on body organs other than the skeleton.

The effects of a hormone depend upon its chemical composition and also upon the characteristics of the location where it is active. The locations of hormonal activity have receptor sites that receive the hormone, like docks receive ships. Receptor sites and their surroundings, like docks and harbors, may vary. The fact that receptor sites vary explains how the same hormone may have different effects in different locations.

Endocrine glands maintain normal baseline levels of hormone; they produce either more or less hormone in response to signals. One signal may be that the hormone level has dropped below its normal baseline, like the thermostat in your house turning on the furnace when the temperature drops too low. A second type of signal is the presence of another hormone whose action stimulates that particular endocrine gland. A change in the level of some body chemical may also be the signal; for example, when blood sugar gets too high the pancreas produces the hormone insulin, which takes sugar into the cells.

Endocrine glands do not respond just to external stimuli, however; they also have internal rhythms. There are regular, cyclic variations in the levels of the hormones. Common cycles are ones that occur about every hour; daily (diurnal) rhythms; and, most familiar, the approximately monthly (trigintal) rhythms. Such natural rhythms make it difficult to be sure that laboratory measurements of a hormone at any one time are truly representative of usual function.

Many very complex chemical processes control bone growth and the maintenance of healthy bone. Several hormones, acting on receptors in the bones, affect those processes. Bone is constructed from materials delivered to it through the bloodstream. Hormones control the blood flow and the concentration of bone-building materials in the blood.

Endocrinology is a young science, and new information about hormonal effects becomes available rapidly. There is still much to know about the effects of hormones on bone. We know some facts about which hormones cause bone breakdown and which stimulate bone formation. Understanding those facts helps us to understand how osteoporosis can be prevented and treated.

The master endocrine gland of the body is the pituitary gland, which is located at the base of the brain. There is a rich blood flow between the base of the brain and the pituitary gland through which pituitary function is influenced by signals from the brain. The hormones produced in the pituitary are effective throughout the body. Pituitary hormones control the production of many of the hormones produced in other endocrine glands, including the thyroid, adrenals, and ovaries.

The pituitary gland produces growth hormone (GH), which influences the growth of bone. Several hormones similar to growth hormone were discovered recently. One function of one of them, prolactin (PRL), is to stimulate the flow of breast milk. Overgrowth of the cells that produce PRL creates small tumors called prolactinomas. People with prolactinomas experience a persistent, milklike discharge from their breasts, a condition known as galactorrhea. Excess PRL, not related to tumors, may occur in response to stress, such as extreme amounts of exercise. Some women who have experienced those changes have also been found to have osteoporosis. The amount of PRL in the blood roughly parallels that of estrogen; PRL levels decrease after menopause and may increase in women who take estrogens. There are many things that we do not yet know about the functions of this recently isolated hormone.

Endocrine glands in the neck influence bone metabolism. The thyroid gland produces hormones that help regulate the speed at which many body processes operate. Excess thyroid hormone causes increased bone breakdown and osteoporosis. Special cell groups within the thyroid produce calcitonin, a hormone that conserves calcium in bone.

Near or within the thyroid gland are tiny glands that regulate blood calcium levels. They are called parathyroid ("para-" means beside) glands, and the hormone they secrete is called parathyroid hormone (PTH), often called parathormone. Muscles and nerves will not function properly unless the calcium concentration of the blood stays within a narrow range. Parathormone secretion is one of the important ways in which the body maintains calcium balance. If the blood calcium level drops, the parathyroid glands produce more parathormone, which mobilizes calcium from the bone storehouses. Excess parathormone, such as may occur from tumors of the parathyroid gland, can cause osteoporosis.

A group of hormones, produced by the testes of men, the ovaries of women, and the adrenal glands of both sexes, are called steroid hormones, or simply steroids. The word "steroid" refers to a chemical configuration shared by many substances. Steroids include sex hormones and a group of hormones similar to cortisone. The steroid hormones help maintain bone. Many of them are used to prevent or treat osteoporosis; others of them cause osteoporosis. There are many different functions of the various steroids, some contrary to one another.

The adrenal glands are located atop the kidneys. The centers of the adrenals produce the hormone adrenaline. The outer layers, the adrenal cortex, produce several hormones. The common name for the best known of the hormones produced by the adrenal cortex is cortisone. A group of substances that share the effects of cortisone are called glucocorticoids, because one of their effects is to increase the amount of sugar (glucose) in the blood. They have potent effects that counteract allergies and the inflammatory reactions of various injuries and diseases. Doctors prescribe synthetic glucocorticoids because of their therapeutic effects. Unfortunately, one severe and frequent side effect of excess glucocorticoids, whether resulting from medicine or disease, is osteoporosis.

The adrenal cortex also produces steroid hormones similar to both female and male sex hormones. Sex hormones help to conserve the strength of bone. So, while the adrenal cortex produces some steroid hormones, the glucocorticoids, which tend to dissolve bone, it produces other steroid hormones that help to conserve bone. Conservation of bone by adrenal hormones becomes especially important for women after the menopause, when their ovaries diminish production of sex hormones. Later in life, at a period sometimes called adrenopause, the adrenal glands cease to be as active. When adrenal function decreases, the effects on bone may vary, although it is generally thought that age-related bone loss slows down at the time of adrenopause.

The hormonal functions of the ovaries are particularly interesting to us because they relate to osteoporosis. The young adult woman's ovaries, which weigh about fifteen grams, are about the size of the end of the thumb. They contain thousands of tiny ova, each with the potential to contribute to a new life. Most of these ova are lost by a withering process called atresia. One ovum each month is dropped into the fallopian tube and makes its way to the uterus. By age fifty the ovaries have shrunk to about one-third the size they were at twenty.

The ovaries secrete hormones that carry on a constant, hormone-communicated dialogue with the pituitary. Each month a pituitary hormone, follicle-stimulating hormone (FSH), stimulates the cells surrounding one ovum to form a follicle that nourishes the ovum. Midway through the menstrual cycle the pituitary abruptly increases production of another hormone, luteinizing hormone (LH). The follicle ruptures and the ovum is passed from the ovary (ovulation) within thirty-six hours after LH reaches a peak level. The empty follicle, called a corpus luteum, secretes large amounts of another hormone, progesterone. Progesterone stimulates the lining of the uterus to accept a pregnancy. If pregnancy does not occur, the production of progesterone abruptly drops, the lining of the uterus sheds, and menstrual bleeding occurs.

During all phases of the menstrual cycle, the ovaries produce hormones called estrogens. Early in the cycle, the main estrogen from the ovary, estradiol, is produced in relatively low amounts. The estradiol level slowly rises to a peak just before the sudden increase in LH from the pituitary. It then falls, only to rise again to a new peak about eight days after ovulation, then falls again if pregnancy does not occur. The peaks and valleys of estrogen levels influence the activities of the pituitary, uterus, and sex organs. Estrogens also have definite, though incompletely understood, effects on bone.

The basic event of menopause is that the cyclic ovarian functions diminish, then cease. Menstrual periods become irregular. Ovulation may occur irregularly even after menstrual periods cease. Estrogen and progesterone production becomes irregular and gradually diminishes. When the pituitary no longer receives cyclic messages from the ovary, it produces excessive amounts of FSH and LH. Though blood tests performed at any one time may not reflect the average situation, the average blood levels of estrogens and progesterone diminish and those of FSH and LH increase during menopause. These events occur more abruptly and profoundly in women who have their functioning ovaries removed—who have a surgical menopause.

Even after the ovaries stop producing estradiol, some estrogens, mostly those known as estrones, are produced from adrenal hormones. Some of the estrones result from a chemical reaction that occurs in body fat. Obese people tend to have more estrogens than thin people, which may explain why overweight women have less trouble with osteoporosis but more worry about cancer of the uterus than thin women. Decreased estrogen production is a major cause of osteoporosis, so women must give serious consideration to estrogen replacement to prevent osteoporosis.

If you are not fascinated by the names of the hormones and the complex interactions described above, don't worry about it. You need not memorize all those facts in order to make reasonable decisions about prevention and treatment. Having read thus far, you have a general idea of how hormones act. The specific information about treatment with hormones is easier to follow.

ESTROGEN TREATMENTS

When women say they are taking hormones, they almost always mean estrogens. There are other hormone treatments for osteoporosis, but we will study estrogen therapy first and in greatest detail. Estrogens have been used longer and studied more closely than any other treatments for osteoporosis.

In 1900, an Austrian gynecologist, Emil Knauer, transplanted ovaries in animals and reversed the symptoms that occurred after the ovaries were removed. By 1917, Stockard and Papanicolaou (for whom the Pap smear is named) had discovered a microscopic method of following the stages of estrus cycles in animals. In Missouri, in 1923, Edgar Allen, a thirty-one-year-old anatomist, and Edward Doisy, a twenty-nine-year-old biochemist, removed liquid from the follicle in a hog's ovary. When they injected the liquid into a mouse whose estrus cycle had been stopped by removal of the ovaries, the mouse's estrus cycle resumed. In 1929, Doisy crystallized the estrogen from that liquid.

Human ovaries produce less estrogen during and after menopause than before. A drop in estrogen level is not the only chemical event that occurs at menopause. There is, however, a strong correlation between estrogen levels and many symptoms of menopause. Estrogen supplements relieve some of those symptoms. In 1940, Fuller Albright suggested that women take estrogens during and after menopause to prevent osteoporosis.

Which women should take estrogens for which symptoms? Variations of that question have stimulated a controversy that has not been resolved over the past five decades. Answers vary in response to medical information, medical opinion, and public sentiment. In the 1960s, women were enthusiastic about taking estrogens to preserve the looks and feelings of youth. Information about possible complications from estrogens caused a reversal of that trend in the 1970s.

Because of the movements for women's rights and consumerism, issues concerning sex hormones are no longer exclusively in the hands of physicians. Physicians receive conflicting mandates from the public, some groups strongly in favor of estrogen therapy and others strongly opposed. Some people regard menopause as a natural event that should not be meddled with, while others regard the symptoms of menopause as a hormone deficiency that should be treated just as one would treat a thyroid deficiency or diabetes. Women who wish to make their own choices about these questions are faced with the same dilemmas that have plagued their physicians.

The questions and information about estrogens are not terribly complex. It is entirely appropriate that laypersons decide whether they and their loved ones should take these drugs. Before you participate in such an important decision, however, you should understand the basic facts about hormones and look at all sides of the issue. Set aside any bias you may have acquired from the opinions of others and look at the facts as they pertain to you. Even after you have done all of that, whether or not to take hormones may still be a difficult decision. You need the counsel of your physician. If you understand the situation and explain your desires, your physician should be able to either assist you in what you have decided or convince you to the contrary.

WHAT ESTROGENS DO FOR YOUR BONES

You cannot decide whether or not you should take estrogens on the sole basis of concern over osteoporosis. However, for many people bone health is the concern that tips the scale in favor of taking them.

Albright recommended that menopausal women take estrogens because he observed that almost all his patients with osteoporosis were postmenopausal women. The severity of osteoporosis depended upon the number of years from menopause more than upon a woman's age. Albright knew that estrogen levels dropped at the time of menopause. There were some, though not many, experimental data to support his hypothesis.

In the twenty-five years after Albright published his findings, many physicians prescribed estrogens to prevent osteoporosis and many others did not. Acceptance of this treatment was widespread but certainly not uniform. Reports about effectiveness were inconsistent. No well-controlled studies had proven

that estrogens were effective treatment for osteoporosis. Bone
health of osteoporotic patients did not improve after administration of estrogens as dramatically as physicians had hoped; many
thought it was no help at all. In 1966, the Food and Drug Administration (FDA) said estrogens were "probably effective" in
the treatment of postmenopausal osteoporosis—a lukewarm, rather
than an enthusiastic, endorsement.

Public opinion and scientific observation of estrogen treatment for osteoporosis collided during the 1970s. Reports that
estrogens cause endometrial cancer and other complications, which
will be discussed later in this chapter, led to closer scrutiny of
the benefits claimed for estrogens. In 1975, action by the Health
Research Group, a consumer advocate organization, led to a court
ruling that any indications for estrogens that had been classed
by the FDA as less than "effective" be removed from the pack-
age inserts. The FDA's advisory committee of endocrinologists
and gynecologists advised that estrogens be regarded as "effective," but it was not until 1981 that their advice was taken.

Ironically, it was at the time the public was expressing greatest
concern over the potential harm of estrogens that well-controlled
clinical studies finally did prove that estrogens help to prevent
osteoporosis in postmenopausal women. A May 1976 article in
the British medical journal *Lancet* stated that it had been proven
that estrogens, taken at the time of menopause, prevent the increasing rate of bone loss that occurs when they are not taken.
By 1979 the National Institutes of Health stated that they recognized the validity of three studies that had shown that bone
loss can be prevented by estrogens taken around the time of
menopause.

In Scotland a double-blind study published in 1980, in which
neither patient nor doctor knew whether estrogen or an inactive
placebo was being taken, showed that over a nine-year period
38 percent of the women who took placebos lost standing height
while only 4 percent of the women who took estrogens became
shorter. A 1980 University of Washington study showed that hip

and wrist fractures were more common among women who did not take estrogens than among women of similar age, income, and education who did take estrogens. A British study in 1982 of one thousand women who took estrogens for an average of over fourteen years showed wrist fracture rates dropped 70 percent below the expected rates and that no hip fractures occurred during the observation period. A 1979 Yale study showed that among women who had fractures, there were relatively few who had taken estrogens. A November 1984 article in the *New England Journal of Medicine* revealed that a study of Mayo Clinic patients showed estrogen deficiency, not aging, was the predominant cause of bone loss that occurred in the first twenty years after menopause.

Now, strong scientific evidence has proven that women who would otherwise rapidly lose bone after menopause and become osteoporotic can retard that bone loss if they take estrogens. More to the point, studies have shown that women who take estrogens to prevent osteoporosis suffer broken hips and wrists and crushed vertebrae far less frequently than women who take no estrogens. In 1983, the Council on Scientific Affairs of the American Medical Association published its conclusion that estrogens effectively prevent osteoporosis.

We do not understand how estrogens protect against bone loss. They may help the intestines absorb more calcium and prevent the kidneys from excreting as much calcium; they may also stimulate the release of the bone-conserving hormone calcitonin. Estrogens may help form liver hormones, which keep cortisone-like steroids from resorbing bone. They may block the effect of the bone-resorbing parathyroid hormone (PTH). They may interact with growth hormone, thyroid hormone, and other hormones that affect bone. In fact, one of the reasons physicians have been reluctant to endorse the use of estrogens for osteoporosis is that the explanations of how estrogens help bone are not adequate.

Estrogens inhibit the breakdown of old bone, but they do

little to stimulate the formation of new bone. Just as clearing condemned buildings may encourage the building of new ones, bone breakdown is one of the things that stimulates bone formation. When breakdown decreases, so does formation. Some studies suggest that people who have already lost bone may regain a small amount if they take estrogens, but there is no firm proof of that. Some women who stop taking estrogens after a number of years may experience rapid loss of bone. Some researchers say those women may end up little better off than they would have had they not taken estrogens at all, but others disagree.

Women who are currently experiencing menopause or who have very recently passed through it have the most to gain from taking estrogens. Those who are otherwise at risk for osteoporosis, as discussed in Chapter 1, have the strongest indications for taking estrogens to preserve bone health. If by taking estrogens you can prevent, or even delay, the rapid loss of bone that occurs at menopause, you may avoid lifelong worry and suffering over fractures.

Since estrogens work best to prevent bone loss and little, if at all, to restore lost bone, benefits from taking them diminish after the rapid bone loss that occurs during and just after menopause. Even if started years after the menopause, however, estrogens still decrease the rate of bone loss, so there is still potential benefit from taking them; it is just that the benefits are greatest if they are begun at the time of menopause.

OTHER BENEFITS OF ESTROGENS

Estrogens were first prescribed in 1931, for the treatment of hot flushes. The exact mechanism of the sweats and flushes that some women experience during the menopause is unknown. When the ovaries decrease production of estrogen and progesterone, the pituitary gland produces increased amounts of the hormones FSH and LH. Production of LH is pulsatile: the peak levels correlate with hot flushes. This is not a complete explanation, however, because women without functioning pituitary glands have experienced hot flushes. Hot flushes can usually be controlled by taking estrogens.

When estrogen levels drop, the skin around the vagina and its inner lining become dry and easily irritated. Sexual intercourse may be painful. Dry skin around the urethra may cause painful urination. Risk of bladder infection increases. Estrogens are effective for the treatment and prevention of vaginal irritation, painful intercourse, and inflammation of the urethra associated with menopause.

Nervousness, depression, anxiety, mood swings, palpitations, headaches, and insomnia are associated with menopause. Whether such symptoms are related to hormonal changes or to some of the psychological adjustments of this time of life is debatable. Whether or not these symptoms are caused by hormonal changes, several well-controlled clinical studies have shown that there are beneficial responses when such symptoms are treated with estrogens. It is more likely that estrogens will be beneficial if these symptoms coincide with hot flushes. Although individual responses vary and symptoms wax and wane regardless of treatment, estrogens seem to relieve many women of these problems.

Premenopausal women have a lower incidence of heart attack than men of the same age. Women who have an early menopause from surgery and do not take estrogen replacements have a higher risk of heart attack than other women of the same age. Those facts led some physicians to prescribe estrogens for men who had had heart attacks. The estrogens did not help prevent further heart trouble in men and may have made things worse. That failure and some studies which linked heart disease to estrogen-containing oral contraceptives have made many people skeptical of the benefits of estrogens for cardiovascular disease. Yet, there are reasons to think estrogens may be of help.

The same one thousand women in the 1982 British study

mentioned above experienced a 63 percent decrease in the expected death rate from heart disease during the fourteen years they took estrogens. Other studies have also shown a decreased incidence of heart-related problems among women who took estrogens after the menopause, but the statistical data are not conclusive enough to confirm that the estrogens were responsible.

Coronary artery disease is correlated with high blood levels of cholesterol molecules called low-density and very-low-density lipoproteins (LDL and VLDL). High-density-lipoprotein molecules (HDL), in contrast, seem to give protection against coronary artery disease. Estrogens cause elevation of the levels of beneficial HDL.

The data presented thus far seem to make a strong case for taking estrogens after menopause. Estrogens protect against osteoporosis, preserve the normal functions of the skin around the vagina, reduce hot flushes, and may help control anxiety and depression and protect against heart disease. There are two things to consider before taking estrogens: one is that the same goals can be approached by some alternative methods, as discussed elsewhere in this book; the other is that there are some serious disadvantages to taking estrogens.

DISADVANTAGES OF ESTROGENS

CANCER OF THE UTERUS The inner lining of the uterus, the endometrium, is a relatively common site of cancer in older women. Each year, about one postmenopausal woman in one thousand will develop endometrial cancer. Endometrial cancer causes about 1.4 percent of cancer deaths in women.

Women who are more than twenty-five pounds overweight develop endometrial cancer about five times as often as thinner women. Women with a family history of uterine cancer and women who have not borne children also have a higher risk of uterine cancer. Of course, women who have had a hysterectomy have no risk for this particular cancer.

Postmenopausal women who have continuously taken estrogens develop endometrial cancer more often than women who have not. That fact has been established by numerous scientific studies. The factor by which the risk is increased has been variously estimated from less than two times to as much as twenty times. Even if the worst were true, the risk of developing endometrial cancer because of estrogen therapy would be quite low, but not low enough to be ignored. The risk of endometrial cancer increases as the duration and the dosage of estrogen therapy increase. Unfortunately, most recent data indicate that prevention of osteoporosis requires prolonged treatment and may be most effective in high dosage. Fortunately, there are some additional, reassuring factors to consider.

Some cancers are much worse than others. The difference depends upon the location, the type of change in the cells, and the speed of detection. Many of the cancers that have resulted from taking estrogens are of a low grade—the cell changes are not extreme and the threat of spread or invasion of surrounding tissues is not great. Since patients taking estrogens are, or at least should be, under medical observation, early detection is more likely for them than for the untreated. Those factors offer some, though not much, reassurance.

What is more reassuring is that women who do not take estrogens continuously and do take them in cycles with progesterone-like drugs (progestogens) seem to have no increased risk for endometrial cancer. Some studies even indicate that their risk of uterine cancer is smaller than that of women who take no hormones at all.

Estrogens stimulate the growth of the endometrium. Continued stimulation of endometrial growth, whether from estrogen pills or from estrogens made by body fat, may cause cancer. In premenopausal women, progesterone changes the endometrial cells and prepares the endometrium for pregnancy. If pregnancy does not occur, progesterone levels drop and the cells are shed during menstruation. Progesterone-like drugs given and withdrawn in cycles help to shed cells that, if left to unopposed estrogen stimulation, might undergo cancerous changes.

Fear of endometrial cancer is one of the several factors to consider before deciding whether to take estrogens. Women who have had a hysterectomy need not worry about cancer of the uterus. Those who do have a uterus have less cause for concern if they can take estrogens in cycles with progestogens. Those who have a uterus and are unable to take progestogens have much more to worry about.

CANCER OF THE BREAST   The breast is the most common site for cancer in women. About one-fourth of all cancer in women is breast cancer, and 20 percent of cancer deaths in women are from breast cancer.

Some women with breast cancers that have spread to other areas seem to improve after their ovaries are removed. Some breast cancers seem to be estrogen-dependent, or have estrogen receptors in them. Normal breast tissue engorges and enlarges when stimulated by estrogens. Those facts and generalized worry about the association of estrogen and cancer have caused concern that estrogens may cause or aggravate breast cancer. However, many studies, some of them of large numbers of patients over many years, show no evidence that estrogens or other hormones cause breast cancer.

Some reports suggest that estrogens, especially when cycled with progestogens, may help reduce the risk or the chance of spread of breast cancer. No one is certain that hormones reduce the risk, but the evidence is strong that estrogens do not increase the risk of breast cancer. Women who have had breast cancer, are currently suspected of having breast cancer, or have a strong family history of estrogen-dependent cancer probably should not take estrogens, but those who have no such history should not base their decisions about taking estrogens upon fear of breast cancer.

STROKES, HEART ATTACKS, AND BLOOD CLOTS   Birth control pills contain estrogens and progestogens. Women who are taking birth control pills have a small increased risk of developing thrombophlebitis, a condition in which the veins develop blood clots that may break loose and lodge in the lungs. Some blood-clotting factors are altered by taking estrogens. Thrombophlebitis occurs more often in older people. Therefore, some people have worried that older people who take estrogens might be increasing their risk of phlebitis.

Observations of large groups of women have shown no increase in the incidence of thrombophlebitis or blood clots among women who take estrogens. In spite of the reassurance from those statistics, however, women who have had thrombophlebitis should consider that as a risk factor when making a decision about estrogen therapy. If the previous episode of thrombophlebitis occurred while taking estrogens or birth control pills, the risk may be greater. Estrogens should probably not be taken when thrombophlebitis is present.

Estrogens may cause some salt and fluid retention. Though not usually a major problem, it could require attention for women who have high blood pressure or have problems with fluid retention. Other diseases that may be made worse by fluid retention, such as migraine and epilepsy, are occasionally aggravated by estrogens. If vision disturbances, headache, or change in mental function occurs while taking estrogens or other hormones, the hormones should be suspected as causes.

GALLSTONES Some groups of women who take estrogens have included more women who developed gallstones than would be expected. Other large studies show no significant correlation between gallstones and estrogen therapy. Some researchers say that women who take estrogens are less likely to develop gallstones. Since there is so much uncertainty and since cholelithiasis (gallstones) is a relatively benign and treatable problem, this factor should not weigh heavily when you decide about estrogen therapy. You should be aware of the possible correlation and alert to the symptoms of gallstones. Gallstones may produce bloating and abdominal pain, usually in the right upper portion of the abdomen. Sometimes the pain will radiate to the right shoulder blade. The symptoms may be associated with nausea and vomiting, and occasionally with jaundice.

VAGINAL BLEEDING Because progestogens theoretically protect against endometrial cancer, it is usually best for women who have not had a hysterectomy to take progestogens if they take estrogens. Later in this chapter there is more information about progestogens. Even though normal menstrual periods may have ceased, some women will experience vaginal bleeding each month for three or four days after they quit taking their progestogen pills. This withdrawal bleeding is usually not as heavy as normal menstrual flow.

For most women, withdrawal bleeding is a nuisance that would not deter them from taking the hormones. However, some women who have fibroids or other causes of excessive or painful bleeding may not be able to tolerate progestogens. Without the safety of progestogens, they may choose to forgo estrogens. Some women have such serious problems with uterine dysfunction that their best choice may be to undergo removal of the uterus. First, however, they should consult with a gynecologist about the indications, risks, and alternatives.

OTHER SYMPTOMS Some women's breasts become tender when they begin taking estrogens; some women experience an increase in sexual desire; about 20 percent of women experience some nausea; and some women feel an increase in appetite.

Such symptoms are not complications; they are merely side effects, which are often transient. If you experience side effects when you first take estrogens, be reassured that they are common, not signs of something gone wrong, and will probably subside spontaneously. You may need to reduce the dosage temporarily, or quit and begin again at a lower dose and increase the dose after you have had time to adjust. The breast soreness may be accompanied by some breast enlargement, similar to breast enlargement during pregnancy, and can be relieved by added support and protection.

Certain laboratory tests, most notably thyroid function tests, are altered by estrogens. Responses to insulin and sugar may change due to estrogens, requiring some adjustment for diabetic women. Pregnant women should not take estrogens or other sex hormones except as specifically directed by a physician who knows about the pregnancy.

ALL RISKS   An all-cause mortality study of over two thousand women from several health centers, coordinated through an agency of the National Institutes of Health, was published in the *Journal of the American Medical Association* in February 1983. It stated that, in women between forty and seventy, the risk of death from all causes was less among women who were taking estrogens than among those who were not. The reasons were not entirely clear, but there were suggestions that there were fewer deaths from cardiovascular disease and that the general life-style and medical care of the estrogen takers may have been better.

Regardless of the reasons for better survival of women taking estrogens, this statistic is reassuring. You can do a lot better for yourself than accepting this one general statistic, though. Consider all of your personal factors as they relate to each of the pros and cons of hormone therapy; consider the alternative and supplemental treatments discussed elsewhere in this book; and consult with your physician before you make a decision.

ESTROGEN TYPES, DOSAGES, AND TREATMENT PLANS

Women should take estrogens only if their ovaries don't produce enough. Symptoms of menopause and decrease in menstruation are the guidelines by which most women judge their estrogen functions. However, women who have had a hysterectomy don't have some of those clues. Women who have had pelvic surgery or other reason for an early menopause may not be able to rely upon the rough guide of being of age for the menopause. Blood tests of hormone levels, microscopic studies of cells from the vagina, or response to a challenge dose of progestogen all may help your doctor advise you whether you are estrogen deficient. Estrogen levels vary even after the menopause, so the values obtained from tests at any one time may not reflect your status at other times and repeated tests may be necessary.

If you know that you are estrogen deficient, if you have weighed the pros and cons of estrogen therapy, and if you have decided that you should take estrogens, you are ready for more decisions. Several different kinds of estrogens are available. You may take them in different ways and according to different dose schedules. You need to decide how long you plan to take them and how you are going to monitor your progress. You must decide what other treatments you are going to coordinate with your estrogen therapy.

You cannot buy estrogens without a prescription. Besides that legal requirement, however, you will want the experience and judgment of a physician who is familiar with these drugs. The physician should help you plan and monitor the course of your treatment. You can best consider all the details as they apply to you. Your physician can best relate your needs to the experiences of others who have had similar needs, monitor your progress, and advise you of new information about these drugs.

The team approach of you and a physician looking out for your interest gives you the best chance of making the right decisions. Do not accept a prescription or refusal of a prescription from a physician who is not willing to discuss this issue with you. If your physician is not comfortable with this problem or if you cannot agree, ask for a referral to a physician with a special interest in this field.

TYPES OF ESTROGENS   If you take estrogens for their general effects, such as treatment of hot flushes or prevention of osteoporosis, it is usual to take them by mouth. Several brands and various chemical preparations are available in small, coated pills that you can take once daily. They are not irritating to the stomach or intestines and are readily absorbed.

When estrogens are taken orally, they are absorbed in the circulation of the intestines and transported to the liver. They alter liver function a little, and the liver makes some changes in the estrogen molecules. If estrogens are not given orally, this first pass through the liver does not occur, although what circulates through the blood eventually passes through the liver. The importance of the changes that occur during the first pass through the liver is not known. Some of the beneficial effects estrogens seem to have on fat metabolism and blood lipids may be lost if this first pass through the liver does not occur.

The word "estrogen" does not refer to a single chemical. Normal body function produces several chemicals with estrogen activity that are, as a group, called estrogens. Commercial preparations include the various naturally occurring estrogens and synthetically made molecules that have estrogen activity. The body reacts to the different preparations in slightly different ways, but there is no one preparation so clearly superior that it is recommended to everyone. The importance of the dose is the effect, not the weight, of the pill, so you cannot judge by the number of milligrams on the prescription. Given what we know now, unless you have found a difference in your personal reactions to various preparations, it is best to take the estrogen preparation your physician recommends.

Estrogen pills are available in several different chemical forms. The dosage schedules quoted in the medical literature usually are for conjugated estrogens (Premarin). "Conjugated" means that a mixture of different, naturally occurring estrogens is blended together. Micronized estradiol (Estrace), ethinyl estradiol (Estinyl), esterified estrogens (Evex, Menest, and Estratab), combined estriol, estradiol, and estrone (Hormonin), chlorotrianisene (Tace), estropipate (Ogen), and quinestrol (Estrovis) are other common oral estrogen preparations manufactured in the United States.

Estrogen also may be administered by vaginal cream. Estrogens are absorbed through the skin and vaginal mucosa. The effects of estrogen-containing creams inserted into the vagina, placed on the skin around the vagina, or rubbed anywhere on the skin are similar to those of oral estrogens. Vaginal administration of estrogens is more effective in lower doses than oral estrogen for the treatment of vaginal drying and irritation around the urethra.

Though the amount of estrogen that is absorbed from creams is unpredictable because of waste and variation in local skin conditions, the same unpredictable absorption also may occur from oral medication because of conditions in the intestines. There is a great deal to learn about which doses and routes of administration of estrogens achieve the various optimal effects of the drug. Information now available confirms that estrogen administered through skin or vagina has substantial general effects, and some physicians believe that vaginal administration is the preferred way to achieve those effects.

Novel ways of slow, predictable absorption of estrogens are being studied. Skin patches similar to nitroglycerin patches used by people with angina are being tested. A reservoir of estrogen is contained between a plastic backing and a control membrane that allows slow diffusion to the skin. Estrogen-soaked vaginal rings have also been tried.

You may also take estrogens by injection. However, since oral and cream preparations are so well absorbed, there is little to recommend injectable estrogens. Subcutaneous pellets that slowly release estrogens were formerly available, but they are not recommended by the FDA at this time because the body tends to form a capsule around the pellet and because there is a constant, rather than the more natural cyclic flow of the drug.

DOSAGE   One response to the concern about cancer was to reassure women that the daily dose of estrogen needed to prevent osteoporosis was lower than the dose given to the women who were found to have an increased incidence of endometrial cancer. Unfortunately, recent information indicates that is not the case, or at least such reassurance must be qualified.

It is not practical here to discuss dosages for all the different estrogen preparations. The points will be illustrated in doses for conjugated estrogens (Premarin) because they are in common use and are often used as the reference in medical reports. It is likely, though not certain, that all the points made here can be translated into equivalent doses of any of the other oral estrogen preparations. Keep in mind that individuals vary in their responses to hormone doses, much more so than for drugs like penicillin or digitalis, which do not occur naturally in the body. Estrogen supplements, unlike those drugs, are added to whatever amount of estrogen is already present in the body.

The lowest dose of conjugated estrogens that causes a decrease in the amount of calcium in the urine is 0.3 mg each day. The lowest daily dose to maintain bone density is 0.625 mg. In some cases, 2.5 mg daily may be necessary to control hot flushes.

Some of the worry about estrogen complications has been stimulated because of complications of oral contraceptives that contain estrogens. Even the low-dose oral contraceptives contain about three times as much estrogen as the dose to maintain bone density. The data on endometrial cancer also suggested that the risk was dose related—the higher the dose, the greater the risk. Thus, the benefit from the relatively low daily dose of 0.625 mg seemed reassuring.

Reassurances about the effective dose being below the high-risk dose must be qualified because of a British study published in the *New England Journal of Medicine* in December 1983. The British doctors began giving women estrogens in 1973. They planned to observe the effect on bone loss. When the risks of estrogen therapy were publicized in the mid-1970s, they reduced the dosages to the minimum necessary to control symptoms of menopause. Study of their results revealed that bone density was maintained best when the women were on the higher doses. Lower doses resulted in less protection against bone loss. At the June 1981 International Symposium on Osteoporosis, in Jerusalem, a San Francisco study team reported that the bone densities of women whose ovaries had been removed were protected from osteoporosis by 0.6 mg but not by 0.3 mg of conjugated estrogens.

Even though higher doses may prevent bone loss more effectively, most women and their physicians prefer the intermediate dose of 0.625 mg daily of conjugated estrogens, or the equivalent of one of the other preparations. That dose seems, at least, to protect the bones and to cause less worry about complications than the higher doses. This is particularly true for the 0.625 mg daily dose if the reason you take estrogens is to prevent osteoporosis and if you take other preventive measures at the same time. You may need higher doses to control hot flushes or other symptoms of menopause or if your bone density decreases while under treatment. Women who also take progestogens or have had a hysterectomy do not have to worry as much about complications.

TREATMENT PLANS The size and chemical composition of the pill you take each day are not the only factors you must consider; you must also select a schedule for taking estrogens and consider the number of years you will take them. Before you begin to take estrogens or other hormones, you should consult with your doctor and plan how long you will take them and what examinations will be necessary before and during your treatment. In most cases, pelvic and breast examinations should be done at the beginning and periodically throughout the treatment. In some cases an endometrial biopsy is done prior to treatment. There are many tests of hormone function. What is important is that you consult with a physician who is alert to the problems and is willing to help you make and adhere to a long-range plan.

Most women who have benefited from taking estrogens have taken them on a cyclic rather than a continuous basis. If you stop taking the pills for a few days each month, you simulate the ebb and flow of your natural estrogen cycle. Complications and side effects are probably reduced by cyclic regimens. Most women find it convenient to take their estrogens every day from the first until the twenty-fifth day of each month and then to stop for the rest of the month. Those who take progestogens coordinate them in this cycle, usually by taking the progestogen from day 16 until day 25.

Since estrogens are easily absorbed and are not irritating, they can be taken at any convenient time of the day. Some women find that side effects such as fluid retention occur less often if they take their estrogen pill at bedtime.

Reliable scientific studies showing that estrogens prevent bone loss have been published recently. Unfortunately, these studies do not give good comparisons that show how long you must take estrogens to protect your bones. We do know that if you begin taking estrogens at menopause and stop after three or four years, you may lose bone rapidly after you stop taking them, delaying the menopausal bone changes for that short time.

If we consider only the effects of estrogen on bone and consider estrogens as the only treatment available, the recommendation would be to take estrogens for life. However, you should consider many other things. Estrogen treatment that is a good idea for an individual at age fifty might not be so at age sixty-five. The decision requires constant reassessment. The important point is that you must take estrogens for a long time if they are to protect your bones from osteoporosis. Treatment plans of less than six years are seldom warranted. Taking estrogens for a few months will not cure osteoporosis or produce any long-range benefit.

MAKING THE DECISION

Do not take the decision for estrogen treatment lightly, especially if you are having symptoms of menopause. Read and reread the above information, but do not base the decision solely on those facts. Prevention of osteoporosis is a major reason for some women to take estrogens. One important thing for you to decide, therefore, is how great is your risk for osteoporosis. Since there are other things you can do to prevent osteoporosis, you must understand those and how they apply to your situation before you can decide how important estrogens are to you. You must understand not only your need and your risks, but also your alternatives; then you need to discuss the matter with your doctor.

There are other hormone treatments for osteoporosis. They are not as practical as some of the nutrition and exercise preventives that we will discuss later, but we will consider the other hormones in this chapter so that we can complete our discussion of hormones. In the summary chapter we will return briefly to the subject of estrogens.

PROGESTOGENS

Just as there are various forms of what are called estrogens, there are several active forms of the progesterone hormones, which are produced by the ovary and the adrenal glands. Synthetically produced drugs with progesterone-like action but slightly different chemical structures are also available. These various natural and synthetic forms are, as a group, called progestogens. Synthetic preparations derived from progesterone are called "progestins." The terminology may be confusing because "progestogen" is sometimes used to refer to synthetics other than progestins and other times the terms are used synonymously. In this book I will use the more general term progestogen and you can assume that the information here applies to any of the drugs called progestins or progestogens.

Progestogens are often taken to protect against the danger of taking estrogens. The normal cycle of ovarian hormone function includes a phase, just after the ovum is passed, when progesterone production rises for several days. One effect of this rise is to prepare the lining of the uterus to accept pregnancy. If pregnancy does not occur, the level of progesterone drops rapidly and menstruation occurs. Without the protective effect of progesterone, the lining of the uterus, the endometrium, is continuously stimulated by estrogen. That is a likely reason that the risk of endometrial cancer is higher in women who take estrogens, but not higher in women who cycle their estrogens with progestogens. Thus, women who have had a hysterectomy have less reason to take progestogens. It may be that a more "natural" sequence of hormone changes occurs when taking both drugs, but the most cogent reason for taking progestogens while taking estrogens, prevention of uterine cancer, is no longer a factor for women who have no uterus.

Progestogens may do more than just protect against the complications of estrogens. Progestogens alone may help prevent osteoporosis. Experimental studies show that receptors in bones that ordinarily bind glucocorticoids, the cortisone-like molecules that may aggravate osteoporosis, may be occupied by progestogen molecules.

At least some of the progestogens may cause a decrease in the level of beneficial high-density lipoproteins (HDL) in the blood. Since people with low HDL levels are more likely to have coronary artery and other cardiovascular problems, progestogens might have an adverse effect on blood vessels.

Worries that progestogens affect blood clotting, thrombophlebitis, hormone-dependent tumors, fluid retention, and change in diabetes control and in some laboratory test values are similar to those about estrogens. In fact, many of the worries stem from experience with women taking both drugs, most especially in the high-dose, combined form of birth control pills. Feelings of depression may occur from taking progestogens.

Synthetic progestogens, such as norethindrone (Norlutin) and norethindrone acetate (Norlutate), and derivatives of natural progesterones such as medroxyprogesterone (Provera, Curetab, Amen) are both prescribed often. Some studies indicate that the beneficial effect that estrogens have on the HDL fraction of blood is maintained better by naturally occurring progestogens. We don't know enough about this, however, and at the present time there does not appear to be any clear advantage of one or the other of these forms of progestogen that would apply to all women.

Progestogens are usually taken for the last seven to ten days of the estrogen cycle, as described above. Such a cycle will cause menstrual bleeding for years beyond what would have occurred naturally. Once such bleeding cycles stop, the need for continued hormone treatment should be reassessed.

As with estrogens, the decision about taking progestogens should be an informed one, based upon the pros, cons, and alternatives. A woman who still has her uterus and who takes estrogens should, under most circumstances, take progestogens too. Whether a woman who does not have her uterus and takes estrogens should take progestogens is controversial. The evidence that progestogens help bone is not strong enough to suggest that women who do not take estrogens should take progestogens just to protect their bones.

ANABOLIC STEROIDS

"Steroids," as we have learned, is a general term that includes many hormones and synthetic substances. Certain steroids may strengthen bone. The steroid hormones that are commonly called "cortisone" weaken bone. Cortisone-like drugs are prescribed so often for the treatment of a great variety of medical disorders that it has become commonplace to use the term "steroids" when referring to cortisone-like drugs.

As if this terminology were not confusing enough, the news contains sensational stories about athletes who take steroids to help build body strength. In this context, steroids refers to a specific group of hormones that stimulate muscle development. Sometimes reporters partially relieve the confusion when they refer to these substances as "anabolic steroids" ("anabolic" means growth stimulating). Because anabolic steroids include and are related to the male sex hormone, testosterone, and have effects that are generally regarded as masculine, they are also called male hormones, or androgens.

Testosterone is produced by the male testes, and, in lesser amounts, by the adrenal glands. Women form small amounts in their ovaries. Many compounds that have anabolic steroid effects are derived, naturally or synthetically, from testosterone. Many brands, either oral or injectable, are available by prescription. Unfortunately, these drugs are also available from illegal sources and are misused by athletes.

Anabolic steroids protect bone from osteoporosis at least as well as estrogens; they may also stimulate new bone formation in a way that estrogens do not. There is no known risk of cancer of the uterus or breast from these drugs; however, other side effects and risks make taking anabolic steroids impractical or inadvisable for most people.

Anabolic steroids have masculinizing effects. They increase facial hair and deepen the voice, and they may cause baldness or acne. Women may experience enlargement of the clitoris when they take these drugs. Paradoxically, some men experience breast enlargement.

Anabolic steroids change liver function tests; therefore, there is concern that they may be harmful to the liver, causing benign tumors and cysts. The HDL fraction of the blood decreases when taking anabolic steroids, so these drugs may contribute to cardiovascular disease. Fluid retention from anabolic steroids may cause high blood pressure, ankle swelling, and other symptoms of excessive fluids.

Because the side effects of anabolic steroids are dose-related, it may be possible to avoid them by low dosage and intermittent use. The ideal dose for the protection of bone is not known, but some investigators have reported that doses within the limits of acceptable side effects have effectively preserved bone. Since many of the side effects are more tolerable to men than to women, anabolic steroids may be a good choice for some men with osteoporosis. Anabolic steroids build muscle as well as bone, so they may be a good treatment for osteoporosis that has developed because of disuse.

Most men who have osteoporosis are old enough to be worried about cancer of the prostate. Since androgens may aggravate cancer of the prostate, men who take these drugs should check with their doctors regularly, and immediately if they notice a change in urination.

CALCITONIN

Calcitonin is produced by specialized cells located in the thyroid gland. Calcitonin conserves calcium in bone, thus acting counter to parathormone, the hormone that mobilizes calcium from bone. Calcitonin levels, which are lower in women than in men, decrease with age; they may increase when estrogens are taken. It would seem, therefore, that calcitonin deficiency might cause osteoporosis, but that has not been proven.

The body responds to calcitonin in some ways that suggest that it helps to prevent osteoporosis. In 1981, researchers from Seattle reported that they had determined from bone biopsies that calcitonin injections had protected their postmenopausal patients from osteoporosis. There are two major problems with calcitonin therapy. One is that effective oral preparations are not available; the other is that antibodies to the injectable preparation, which is derived from salmon, appear in the blood after about six months of therapy.

GROWTH HORMONE

The pituitary gland produces growth hormone. Since growth hormone makes young bones grow, there is reason to think it might make grown bones stronger. There are many derivatives and variations of growth hormone, but there are no effective oral preparations. We do not know enough about the various types and effects of the growth hormone–like substances. Research in this area could lead to an effective treatment for osteoporosis.

OTHER HORMONE TREATMENTS

Hormones that are ordinarily considered to make osteoporosis worse are sometimes prescribed for treatment of osteoporosis. The idea is to stimulate new activity in bone, like tearing down an old building in hopes that someone will build a new and larger one. Thyroid, glucocorticoid, and parathyroid hormones are examples of hormones so used during short-term or intermittent periods in conjunction with other drugs. These hormones are prescribed for osteoporosis only in research or carefully controlled clinical situations. Insulin may have some positive effect on bone strength, but its other effects are too potent to permit its use for people other than diabetics.

6

Nutrition for Strong Bones

MOST PEOPLE know that growing bones require healthful food. Not everyone knows what eating habits are best for growing children, however, and not everyone knows how important nutrition is to bones after growth ceases.

People are not ignorant about nutrition because they don't care, but because they receive a great deal of conflicting and erroneous information. Some of the faulty information is the result of outdated knowledge, some is from seemingly well-reasoned but ultimately unfounded theory, and some is the result of commercial exploitation. However, while there are still things to be learned, modern knowledge of nutrition does provide clear guidelines to what foods you should eat for healthy bones and general good health.

The need for good bone-building materials never ends, since bones constantly resorb and reform themselves. Bones stop growing only in the sense that they don't get longer; otherwise, they grow throughout life. The foods bones need to maintain health are similar to those that support growing bone. Only a few things that people eat are directly harmful to bone, although many diet excesses cause poor general nutrition, which indirectly destroys bone.

Since this book is about bones, the first discussions in this chapter are about what your bones need from your diet. Good general health is essential to good bone health, and diet advice that focuses on only one aspect of health is not good diet advice; so, following the examination of what bones need, general recommendations about diet are made. I have given the most complete information about those aspects of diet that are important to your bones, but some of the recommendations are more related to general health. We will also examine the particular dietary needs and problems of special groups of people: the young, the old, the poor, the rich, vegetarians, the overweight, and the underweight.

WHAT BONES NEED

CALCIUM   As we have seen, calcium is extremely important in maintaining strong bones. Calcium is a silver-white metal. Few people are used to thinking of calcium as a metal because, in nature, it almost always exists in combination with other ions. Calcium is very abundant in nature, especially in marble, limestone, sand, and in internal skeletons (bones) and external skeletons (shells) of animals.

Calcium is the dominant element in human bone. The body contains about 1.3 kg (about 3 pounds) of calcium. Even though the calcium in blood and other body fluids is critical to life, 99 percent of your body's calcium is in your teeth and bones.

It is not enough to consume 3 pounds or so of calcium during the years of childhood growth and not worry about it thereafter. Each day you lose calcium in urine, feces, and sweat. If you don't replace what you lose, your bones suffer. The amount of calcium you lose varies with your age, health, activities, and other things in your diet. The average person loses more than 500 mg of calcium each day. Even if you knew exactly how much calcium you lost each day, you would not know how much calcium to eat. Not all the calcium you eat is absorbed; some passes right on through and does you no good. Therefore, you must take in more than you lose. That is a safe practice, because a little excess calcium is not harmful: your intestines and kidneys pass off what your bones do not need.

Scientists who recommend how much calcium you should have in your diet account for variations in need, incomplete absorption, and the safety of reasonable excess. The idea of a "minimum daily requirement" (MDR) has largely been replaced by the more practical concept of a "recommended daily allowance" (RDA). In the United States, RDAs (or USRDAs) are determined about every five years by the Food and Nutrition Board of the National Academy of Sciences and the National Research Council.

In the past, the official RDA for calcium was 800 mg. In light of recent knowledge about osteoporosis, that figure is probably too low. It is certainly too low for growing children, pregnant or nursing women, and women during and after the menopause.

Osteoporosis develops so slowly and has so many causes that it has been difficult for scientists to assign a daily calcium intake requirement that would account for the needs of those who may get osteoporosis. One study, done in Yugoslavia in 1979, showed that people who lived in a region where their dietary calcium was about 950 mg per day had higher bone-mineral contents than ethnically similar people who lived in a nearby area where the daily dietary calcium was about 450 mg per day.

Adolescents need 1,500 mg of calcium daily. Pregnant and nursing women should receive at least 2,000 mg of calcium in their diets; 2,500 mg for pregnant or nursing adolescents. During and after menopause women should have 1,500 mg of calcium in their daily diets. Since older people do not absorb calcium as well as younger people, the daily requirement for men should increase with age, probably to about 1,000 mg. That leaves a relatively small group of young, adult, non-childbearing people whose bones may be adequately served by 800 mg of calcium per day.

At the risk of boring you with repetition, I keep saying "daily" or "per day." Taking in 2,000 mg of calcium one day, and none the next, does not maintain healthy bone as efficiently as taking in at least your daily requirement every day. If you have a mason building a brick wall for you, the way you have osteoblasts building bone for you, it is best to keep the mason supplied with bricks and mortar. A mason can only build so fast, so extra materials don't help; if he runs out of materials, progress on the wall suffers. Like most building jobs, the storage space for extra materials is limited, so fresh supplies are needed on a regular basis. And while a little extra calcium cannot hurt you, no one has shown any practical or theoretical benefit to taking more than 1,500 mg of calcium a day, except for pregnant or nursing women, and there may be some ill effects from such a practice.

Details about the calcium content of various foods are included in the information about healthful diets later in this chapter. Calcium is one of the few food substances that may, in some circumstances, best be taken as a pill. Discussion of calcium pills is included in Chapter 7.

PHOSPHATES   Phosphates are combinations of phosphorus and oxygen with other elements. Bone mineral has a high phosphate content. Measurable phosphate levels, such as those in blood, seem to parallel bone growth, since they are higher in infancy and adolescence. Many researchers think that phosphates are very important to bone formation and maintenance, but the positive aspects of dietary phosphates are not well understood. There may be circumstances when more phosphate is needed for bones, but, if there are, they have not been defined.

Most information about dietary phosphate is negative—that is, it describes the harmful effects of excess phosphate. Phosphate absorption and metabolism are very closely linked to calcium. Phosphate excess interferes with the absorption of calcium. If the body content of phosphate is too high, the body's efforts to rid itself of excess phosphates may result in calcium loss. Food additives, soft drinks, and red meats are phosphate rich, so the diets of most people in developed societies contain more than enough phosphate.

Present information suggests that there is very little indication to supplement your diet with phosphates. There are good reasons to avoid excessive phosphate intake, however, especially if your calcium intake is marginal. If you have and are going to maintain a high phosphate diet, you should consider your need for calcium to be greater than normal and adjust your calcium intake accordingly.

PROTEIN One of the most widely held myths about nutrition is that we must take great care to get enough protein. In areas of great poverty and lack of agricultural resources, inadequate dietary protein produces dramatic starvation diseases. Some people have supposed that the opposite must be true, that extraordinarily high protein diets would produce extra-good health. Later in this chapter, the section about healthy diets will dispel that myth and explain the harm excessive protein may bring to your general health.

The basic material of bone, upon and within which the mineral crystals reside, is collagen. Collagen is composed of interconnected molecules of amino acids, which are fragments of protein. The body can create some amino acids, but others must come from protein in the diet. Therefore, it is necessary to the health of bone that there be an adequate amount of protein in your diet. Protein can be stored fairly well, so a steady stream of dietary protein may not be as important as a continuous supply of calcium.

High-protein diets cause people to lose more calcium in feces and urine. Osteoporosis is more common in parts of the world and among peoples who have a great deal of protein in their diets. Experiments show increased rates of resorption and reformation of the underlying matrix of bone and decreased rates of mineral deposition when animals are fed high-protein diets.

An adequate and reasonable amount of protein is important

to bone health and general health. Dietary protein is especially important during growth, although it is also important that growing children learn to avoid the excesses that may accompany high-protein diets. Some protein-rich foods are harmful to general health, and excess protein in the diet may cause you to lose calcium and may weaken your bones.

TRACE ELEMENTS   Besides calcium, many other elements are important to healthy bone. The precise effects and the exact amounts needed are not completely understood. Because the obvious factor they have in common is that they are present in very small amounts, they are often lumped together in a category called "trace" elements, meaning that in gross chemical analysis only traces of them are present.

On food and supplement labels, trace elements are sometimes called "minerals." They usually do exist as minerals, meaning they are usually in combination with other elements. Since the body usually breaks up those combinations and frees the individual element to combine in other ways, it is best to consider the elements individually.

Fluorine, in its uncombined form, is a gas similar in many ways to chlorine. The element fluorine exists in liquid and solid materials as the ion fluoride, often combined with other ions or attached to complex crystals like those in bone. When people speak of this element, as they often do because of its well-known role in the prevention of tooth decay, they usually speak of "fluorides."

There are some good reasons to think that fluorides may be very important to bone health. Scientific study has left little doubt that fluorides help teeth stay healthy. There are many similarities between the chemistry of teeth and bones. Some, though not all, studies of populations in high- and low-water-fluoride areas have shown more problems with osteoporosis in the low-fluoride areas. Most impressive are the data in the next chapter about the ways in which high-dose fluoride supplements strengthen weak bone.

It will be a long time before we know whether or not low-dose fluoride supplements will do anything to prevent osteoporosis. A 1966 study in North Dakota showed that people in an area of high-fluoride water had more mineral in their spines than people where the water fluoride content was low.

Another study, done by researchers at the National Center for Health Statistics and the National Institute on Aging, compared statistics about death from hip fractures and fluoride content in drinking water. They found that people in areas of high-fluoride content had lower death rates from hip fractures, but only in areas where the fluoride content was higher than that ordinarily recommended to prevent tooth decay.

Some studies show little correlation between water fluoridation and osteoporosis. Data are accumulating, and public health scientists are interested in the relationship between fluoride consumption and osteoporosis. There are many variables to contend with, and the observation periods must be very long.

Dentists are way ahead of physicians in advising people about fluoride. If your drinking water contains less than 0.7 ppm (parts per million), the chance of tooth decay is much greater. Information about the fluoride content of your drinking water should be available from your local health department or your water supplier. Only about 5 percent of Americans have adequate natural fluoride in their drinking water, but over half drink water that has been supplemented with enough fluoride to help prevent tooth decay.

At this time we don't know what amount of fluoride is ideal for bones; at what age fluoride supplementation should begin, if at all; how many years fluoride supplementation should be continued and at what level; or what the dangers of supplements in excess of those recommended for tooth decay might be. If your drinking water contains less than 1 ppm of fluoride, you should probably take one to four of the 2.2-mg sodium-fluoride tablets usually recommended for prevention of tooth decay. The dose would depend upon how fluoride-deficient your water is.

However, do not assume that if a little fluoride is good, more is better. High doses of fluoride can be very dangerous, even lethal. As you will read in Chapter 7, fluoride in moderately high doses has been used to treat osteoporosis, but you should never try to do that yourself. If you take higher doses, do so only under the management of and in careful compliance with the recommendations of a physician who is familiar with the use of fluorides as a drug.

Magnesium is a metal that gets relatively little attention for its role in human function. It is not present in high concentration in any one body tissue, yet it is the body's fourth most abundant metal (after sodium, potassium, and calcium). Although it is best known for its importance to muscle contraction, 65 percent of the body's magnesium is contained in bone.

Magnesium is chemically similar to calcium in many ways. Magnesium deficiencies result in impaired growth and low levels of serum calcium; excessive magnesium is associated with loss of bone minerals.

Present knowledge suggests that, except in the presence of unusual disease states, some poisonings, and very unusual diet practices, too much or too little magnesium is seldom a factor in human disease. The effects of prolonged minor magnesium deficiency or excess on bone are unknown.

Zinc is another metal essential to health, although in very small amounts. More zinc is present in bone than in other tissues. Zinc has been found to concentrate along the surfaces where new bone is forming. People who are zinc-deficient have wounds that are slow to heal, and some experiments suggest that zinc supplements may speed healing. Therefore, zinc may be important to bone health, but we do not know the long-term effects of too much or too little zinc on bone.

Other elements present in tiny amounts in bone include copper, potassium, sodium, iodine, chromium, sulfur, manganese, and molybdenum. Potassium and sodium are so abundant in the body that they cannot be considered trace elements, but they are in such relatively low concentrations in bone that their roles in bone are either not very important or our present knowledge is not adequate for us to understand their importance.

The trace elements are discussed further in the section on healthy diet. For most trace elements, we have no more than hints of their importance. We know that some of these elements in our diets are necessary, but we also know that most diets provide what appears to be enough of all of them (except for fluorides in fluoride-deficient-water areas). We know that there are similarities and interrelationships between some of these elements, so that excess of one may lead to deficiency of another.

We do not know enough about the trace elements to make exact recommendations, but we do know which foods contain them. If your diet is deficient in those foods, you may want to take supplements in low doses, but in our present state of ignorance it seems dangerous to take large amounts.

VITAMINS In 1753, James Lind, a Scottish naval surgeon, proved that sailors who ate limes did not get scurvy. Scurvy causes the gums and teeth to go bad and results in unhealthy blood vessels and supportive tissues. After Lind's discovery, British sailors always had limes available; hence they were called "limeys." The scurvy-preventing ingredient in limes proved to be ascorbic acid, or vitamin C. From that time, medical science has searched for other vitamins. The current count is thirteen.

Vitamins are needed in trace amounts. They are not called trace elements because they are not elements. They are organic molecules, meaning that they are carbon-containing molecules, chemically more complex than the simple elements discussed above. All of the thirteen vitamins are essential to health. The total amount of all of them needed each day for a week would not fill a teaspoon.

Vitamin D is particularly important to bone. Without vitamin D, the body cannot absorb adequate amounts of calcium from the food in the intestines. Vitamin-D deficiency during growth causes characteristic bone deformities called "rickets"; vitamin-

D deficiency in adults causes osteomalacia. Osteomalacia may coexist with osteoporosis, and it may be hard to distinguish the effects of the two problems. Because of that overlap, there is some controversy about whether a minor vitamin-D deficiency may cause plain, idiopathic osteoporosis. Since vitamin-D deficiency impairs calcium absorption and since calcium deficiency is a cause of osteoporosis, it seems likely that vitamin-D deficiency contributes to osteoporosis, even in the absence of obvious osteomalacia.

The distinction between osteoporosis and osteomalacia may become important when a doctor decides whether or not to use vitamin D in high doses, as a drug, but it is not important to you when you decide what diet or diet supplements are important to maintain bone health. Vitamin D in low doses is harmless and essential to healthy bone; in high doses it is dangerous and must be carefully managed by a physician.

The recommended daily allowance of vitamin D is 200 IU (international units) for adults and 400 IU for children. Vitamin D is fat soluble, so it is stored if taken in excess. Much excess can be quite dangerous, even life-threatening. Excess vitamin D may also be contraproductive to the improvement of bone health. Vitamin D stimulates bone breakdown, so if taken in excessive doses, it could make osteoporosis worse.

Vitamin D occurs in different forms. Some vegetable matter contains ergocalciferol, which, like the more common animal form, cholecalciferol, can be converted by the liver and kidneys to the active form of vitamin D. Fifteen to sixty minutes of sunlight each day will change a skin component, 7-dehydrocholesterol, into vitamin D. Vitamin-D deficiencies may be caused by one or some combination of diet deficiencies, inadequate exposure to sunlight, or abnormalities in the kidneys or liver. People with adequate sun exposure or healthy diets need not worry about vitamin-D deficiency unless they have kidney disease, liver disease, or some problem with vitamin-D metabolism. People who are vitamin D–deficient because of one of those diseases usually need vitamin D in high doses and may require special, "activated" forms of vitamin D.

Vitamin C is important to the health of tissues containing a great deal of collagen. Collagen is the basic protein structure of bone. Acute deficiency of vitamin C, scurvy, causes such severe effects to the rest of the body that any effects on bone are not apparent; that is, the other symptoms may become severe before noticeable changes in bone have time to develop.

Whether or not marginally low vitamin-C intake over a long time could result in damage to bone, while never causing the obvious symptoms of scurvy, is unknown. It is also not known whether certain people need more vitamin C than others and manifest their needs only by subtle changes that would not ordinarily be attributed to vitamin-C deficiency. It is possible, though entirely unproven, that a slowly developing process of loss of collagen-containing tissue, like osteoporosis, could be related to a vitamin deficiency.

RDAs are usually two to six times the MDRs. The MDR is the level below which symptoms appear. RDAs are determined from the best available contemporary knowledge by scientists who know what they are doing. If the symptoms of a deficiency are not recognized, scientists do not know how to establish either the MDR or the RDA.

Some recommendations for very large doses of vitamins are based upon the belief that symptoms of the deficiency state have not been properly recognized. There are possibilities that such beliefs might someday prove true. Until some proof is available, however, it is best to regard benefits from high doses of C or other vitamins as rather remote hopes for future developments in the quest for bone health.

FOODS DESTRUCTIVE TO BONE

Excesses of some trace elements and vitamins can cause loss of the mineral content of bone. Magnesium and vitamin D were mentioned previously. Vitamin A in excess is very dangerous. Among the effects of vitamin-A excess are loss of bone mineral. The source of most such excesses is ill-advised self-treatment with large doses of over-the-counter vitamins and minerals, since only very unusual diets would produce significant excess of vitamins and minerals. An example is the diet of some Eskimos, who consume huge amounts of vitamin A–saturated walrus livers.

The common source of dietary destruction of bone is alcohol. Alcohol reduces intestinal absorption of calcium and interferes with calcium and zinc metabolism. It provides empty calories that interfere with good general nutrition. Alcohol causes irritation of the stomach, which is often soothed by antacids containing aluminum, which further interfere with calcium absorption. Coffee and highly spiced foods may also be indirectly destructive to bone because they lead to the ingestion of antacids.

WHAT IS A HEALTHY DIET?

LOW IN SATURATED FATS In 1977, George McGovern chaired the U.S. Senate Select Committee on Nutrition and Human Needs. Like most government investigations, the conclusions of this committee were based not upon the cutting edge of scientific progress but upon evidence that had been apparent to doctors and scientists for a long time. McGovern's committee reported that arteriosclerosis, heart disease, high blood pressure, stroke, diabetes, and some cancers were all related to the American diet. They recommended that Americans eat less animal fat, processed food, sugar, salt, and alcohol, and fewer calories. Many people regard such reports as government intrusion on the fun in life, but the government only collected the conclusions. The facts came from objective physicians and scientists who had observed human suffering for many years.

When I was in medical school in the early 1960s, I was taught that the fats contained in butter, eggs, whole milk, red meats, and some shellfish caused an increase in the amount of fat and cholesterol in the blood. Such fats are called "saturated," referring to a characteristic of the chemical bonding in the fat molecules. Unsaturated fats, such as those in most vegetable oils, did not seem to cause the same trouble.

We also knew that high blood fat and cholesterol were characteristic of patients who suffered heart attacks, strokes, and other diseases related to the buildup of the fatty, arteriosclerotic plaque we saw on the insides of arteries in the pathology lab. It is too bad that everyone does not have the opportunity to see how those plaques fill up the insides of arteries. If they could, they would take the warnings of the McGovern Committee and others more seriously.

Young people think of themselves as being immortal. They do not feel the effects of slowly progressive diseases that will damage them in middle life. They tend to ignore advice about such things as proper diet. Even in the early sixties we knew that autopsies done on American victims of the Korean War had shown significant buildup of ugly plaque in the coronary arteries of 35 percent of twenty-two-year-old soldiers.

Unfortunately, only a few lucky people believed the reports back in the fifties and sixties and changed their diets accordingly. Over the years since, more people have come to believe those reports, but often they give them little serious consideration until their attention is caught by a heart attack or another such complication. As of the writing of this book, news releases about research confirming the correlation between a high-fat diet and cardiovascular disease are still treated like new information.

Diets that are low in saturated fats do not have to be tasteless. Diets low in animal fat do not have to be low in calories. Such diets do not require that you give up the ingredients of milk and protein-containing foods that are important to the health of your bones.

One aspect of American life that has been almost as dear to our culture as the automobile has been the consumption of large quantities of red meat. The steak is a symbol of affluence and celebration. The standard American breakfast is bacon or sausage and eggs. American kids grow up on hamburgers. We call our food our bread and butter. With the exception of bread, every one of those foods is rich in harmful fats.

We have been indoctrinated with the idea that we need large quantities of protein and that we must get that protein from meat, eggs, and whole milk. However, our need for protein has been greatly exaggerated: six or seven ounces of meat, chicken, or fish provide enough protein for a one-hundred-fifty-pound person for one day.

The media do not provide enough information about obtaining adequate protein from nonanimal sources. Two-thirds of the protein ingested by Americans comes from animal sources; if it were one-third, the United States would be a much healthier nation. Many nations in northern Europe are just as bad; statistics about animal fat consumption in Finland are even worse than those in the United States. The problem is not so much that animal protein is bad as that animal proteins are often rich in saturated fats.

Fish, except for shellfish, and chicken, except for the skin, are excellent sources of protein. They are not high in fat unless they are fried or otherwise prepared in a fatty sauce. Beans, soybeans, rice, whole grains, and skimmed milk are other low-fat sources of protein.

LOW SUGAR The average American eats one hundred twenty-eight pounds of sugar each year, about one-third of a pound every day. About six hundred calories each day are consumed as simple sugars. Besides what we sprinkle on our food, we preserve and alter the taste of almost all processed foods with sugar. Few ingredients labels do not list sugar, dextrose, glucose, fructose, or sucrose. An eight-ounce soft drink contains about six teaspoonfuls of sugar. Do not kid yourself about honey and "natural" sugars—it is all simple sugar contributing the same problems to a healthy diet.

Sugar in itself is not dangerous, except to people with diabetes. The problem with simple sugars is that they are rapidly absorbed, result in a rapid rise in blood sugar, and give a transient feeling of satisfaction. There follows a rapid drop in blood sugar, with a feeling of hunger and discontent. When we then try to satisfy that uneasy feeling by eating more simple sugars, the cycle begins again. The net effect is a diet that is high in calories and low in nutrition.

LOW SALT   The other common excess in the American diet is salt. The average American consumes about fifteen pounds of salt each year, or about three teaspoonfuls per day. We need some salt—about one-tenth of one teaspoonful per day. We get thirty times as much as we need and take in about three times the maximum we should allow ourselves. High blood pressure is ten times as common among people who consume a lot of salt. Many people can bring their high blood pressure into the normal range simply by limiting their salt intake.

If you do sprinkle salt on food, you are almost surely getting too much salt. The taste for heavily salted food is an acquired habit. Once you break it, excessively salty food will no longer taste good to you.

You do not have to sprinkle salt on food to get too much salt. Processed foods are loaded with salt. Canned vegetables may contain one hundred times as much salt as fresh vegetables. Most breads and crackers are rich in salt.

By now, you are probably thinking that you are back where you started; your bones need all sorts of nutrients, but practically all food is bad for your general health. However, there are good things you can eat to give you all the nutrition you need, even more than you need if you want to gain weight. There are good things to eat that will provide your bones with all they need.

You may be surprised to learn that one of the best ways to achieve good bone and general nutrition is with the oldest diet staple in the book—milk.

MILK   Milk is available in many different forms. Whole milk contains over 3.25 percent fat, which is too much. Lowfat milk contains between 0.5 and 2 percent fat. Skim, or nonfat, milk contains less than 0.5 percent fat. Skim milk has every bit of the calcium and protein of whole milk.

Evaporated milk has about 60 percent of the water removed; it may be either whole or skim. Buttermilk, unlike the name suggests, is lowfat or nonfat milk to which bacteria have been added to ferment the sugars. Cream and sour cream contain over 18 percent milk fat. Heavy cream, or whipping cream, contains over 38 percent fat.

Most milk is fairly high in salt (about 120 mg of sodium per cup), but low-sodium milk, with about 95 percent of the sodium removed, can be purchased. For those who want fat in their milk but want to avoid saturated fats, "filled" milk has had the milk fat removed and replaced with vegetable fats.

Although milk is a good source of bone nutrients, some people cannot tolerate it, because it gives them abdominal cramps or diarrhea. The most common reason for this is intolerance of lactose, one of the sugars in milk. However, acidophilus milk, which has had the lactose predigested, is available, although the taste is slightly different. Sweet acidophilus milk contains bacteria that digest the lactose only after it is warmed in your body. Some people can tolerate regular milk if they take lactase powders or tablets.

Yogurt is milk that has been treated with bacteria. The lactose content of yogurt is low, and many people who cannot tolerate milk can enjoy yogurt. Yogurt can be made from milk with or without fat: the label will tell you the fat content.

CALCIUM   One cup of whole milk contains 288 mg of calcium. Actually, skim milk contains slightly more—296 mg. One cup of yogurt contains about the same amount, as does an ounce of Swiss cheese, an ounce and a half of cheddar cheese, two cups of cottage cheese, or a little less than two cups of ice cream. Powdered nonfat milk, which contains 50 mg of calcium per teaspoonful, can be used as an additive in baking, coffee, dressings, and sauces.

Many other foods contain calcium. None contain calcium in the amount and the available form that milk and related dairy products provide. Broccoli, mustard, collards, spinach, rhubarb, and turnip greens are calcium rich, but they contain oxalates that may interfere with the ability to absorb calcium. Almonds and tofu are high-calcium foods. Oysters, salmon, and sardines are high in calcium, but tuna, crab, haddock, and many other seafoods are not.

Bones, of course, are high in calcium. If you put a little vinegar in soup stock you can leach the calcium out of the soupbone, then boil it for a while to boil off the vinegar; the calcium will remain in the soup.

Unless your diet is very rich in some of these other calcium-containing foods, you will need to ingest about four cups of milk or equivalent dairy products each day, in addition to what calcium you get from other foods, to get 1,200 to 1,500 mg of calcium daily. That may be the best way, but many people find that impractical. If you cannot or will not do it, then you should take calcium pills as described in the next chapter.

BULK   In the 1970s researchers in the United Kingdom noted that people with plenty of fiber in their diets had less bowel disease, including less cancer of the colon and rectum. Fiber means cellulose and other plant components that are not absorbed by the human intestines. Fruits, leafy vegetables, raw carrots, and whole grains like bran are rich in fiber. Many cereal and bread labels contain information about fiber content. Such fibers increase the volume of feces; thus, diets rich in fiber are called bulk diets.

Bulky, fiber-filled stools carry some important nutrients away with them. For example, the amount of calcium lost in the stool increases with high-bulk diets. Bulky stools also cause increased loss of zinc, iron, phosphorus, magnesium, copper, and water.

In spite of the losses that may occur, a healthy diet should have a high fiber content. The decreased risk of large-bowel cancer and other colon diseases is worth correcting any losses that occur. Bulk diets may help decrease cholesterol because they stimulate excretion of cholesterol-rich bile. High-bulk diets usually relieve constipation problems. They are preferable to the consumption of laxatives, which probably cause more problems with loss of nutrients than bulk diets.

If you have not been on a high-fiber diet before, do not begin one abruptly. Slowly increase the amounts of fiber-rich foods in your diet. Be sure you consume adequate amounts of calcium and the other minerals mentioned, since you will begin losing slightly greater amounts in your stool. Also increase your consumption of fluids. Skim milk and bran cereals with fruit make a good meal that provides fiber and most of the correction you need for the extra bulk.

MINERALS AND VITAMINS   Calcium is the mineral component you need to worry most about when you adjust your diet to provide for bone health. Calcium sources were described above in the discussion of milk. Milk is a very complete food, but it does not contain adequate amounts of iron, manganese, copper, or vitamin C. The potato is another well-rounded food, if eaten with its skin.

A balanced diet of milk, fresh fruits, leafy green vegetables, yellow vegetables, potatoes, whole grains, and lowfat meats will provide you with all the nutrients you need. You may not get enough fluorides if your water is fluoride deficient, but tea, fish, and many animal foods contain fluoride. If you live where the water is "hard," you are more likely to be getting more trace elements (and a little extra calcium) than if your water is soft or highly purified.

If you eat a truly healthful diet every day, supplements probably will not help at all. Mineral and vitamin supplement pills are often justified because few people are organized and disciplined enough to stay on a healthful diet all the time. Processed and commercially prepared foods may lose their natural vitamins and minerals.

RDAs for vitamins and minerals are determined for all people over age fifty as a group. People over sixty-five may absorb less than those between fifty and sixty-five and, therefore, require more vitamins and minerals in their diets than suggested by current RDAs. They should consider their RDAs to be slightly but not grossly higher than published values.

If you have a special health problem that increases your need for vitamins and minerals, if there are reasons that you cannot maintain a well-rounded, healthy diet, or if you want to concentrate on other aspects of diet health and not worry about vitamin and mineral deficits, then you should take a supplement. Many people, for one of those good reasons, take vitamin and mineral pills. That does not explain how the vitamin pill business has become a $1.5-billion-a-year industry in the United States. Rather, vitamin pills are a huge business in the United States and elsewhere because people take excessive amounts of vitamins and minerals unnecessarily. Usually nothing is harmed except the pocketbook; the excesses are merely not absorbed or are rapidly excreted in the urine. However, the fat-soluble vitamins A, D, and K are stored in body fats and may more readily concentrate to toxic levels; even usually harmless vitamin C causes nausea and diarrhea when taken in excess.

Vitamin D is present in fortified milk, egg yolk, liver, tuna, salmon, and cod-liver oil; it may also be derived from sunshine. Excess vitamin D can cause kidney stones, nausea, deafness, high blood pressure, and high cholesterol. Although you are not likely to get excess vitamin D from food or sunshine, do not take vitamin-D supplements without a doctor's prescription.

Many people take high doses of vitamins or minerals because they have tried to analyze their own symptoms, then looked for popular explanations and corrections. The vitamin and health faddist industries are all too willing to provide those explanations and to encourage the consumption of large quantities of pills.

There is some chance that medical science has not recognized the benefits of very high doses of some vitamins, although it is not because no one has been researching it. A great deal of study has been done to determine the effects of different doses of vitamins and minerals, and that research is the basis of the recommended daily allowance. But no one claims we know it all, so the possibility exists that there are unrecognized benefits of high doses of vitamins and minerals.

Before you take the advice of someone selling vitamin and mineral supplements or decide, on your own, to take high doses of some vitamin or mineral, consider a corollary of the logic in the previous paragraph. If there is a possibility that medical science is unaware of some benefit from high doses of a vitamin or mineral, there is also a possibility that there exists some unrecognized harm from such doses.

Vitamins and minerals exist in adequate proportion in a healthy diet. If your diet is not always ideal, you can safely supplement it by taking a vitamin and mineral pill in roughly the proportions available in a healthy diet. That way you are following Mother Nature's prescription, which also happens to approximate the prescription of well-studied research. Do not take vitamins and mineral supplements in excess of your RDA.

Synthetic vitamins are cheaper and more pure than "natural" vitamins. If you get your vitamins and minerals the natural way (from food), that is fine, but do not waste money on "natural" pills or powders. It may seem like a good idea to take ground-up bonemeal or other combinations that sound natural, but you are less certain of getting what you really need and there is some worry about ingesting harmful impurities, such as lead. If you want a vitamin supplement, take it in the morning with your meal to get maximum absorption.

SPECIAL DIET PROBLEMS

CHILDREN Parents have a difficult time providing good nutrition for their children, since children are not responsive to long-term worries about the effects of diet on health. Instead, they are responsive to the blitz of commercials and social pressures that persuade them to follow atrocious dietary habits.

Not many children are impressed with the fact that they are building a bone bank from which they will make withdrawals as they pass through life, and that if their bank is not well endowed in childhood, their bones will break when they get old. They should learn those facts, but telling them those things is not enough to protect them from the undermining influences of pop culture.

The soft drink and hamburger industries are enormous. They depend upon selling bad nutrition to children. Fast-food hamburgers and hot dogs are high in harmful fats, low in fiber, low in vitamins, high in salt, and very expensive for what little nutrition they contain. Of all the fad and fast foods with mass appeal to the young, only pizza has the potential for reasonable nutritive value. Pizza made with pre-prepared and processed ingredients and loaded with fatty meat additives is bad nutrition, but it does not have to be made with harmful ingredients. Bread, cheese, tomato sauce, and vegetable toppings may be quite nutritious if the ingredients are fresh and of good quality.

Children should drink at least thirty-two ounces of milk each day. Skim milk is best, but if they will not drink it, lowfat milk is not bad. Do not get them into the whole-milk, animal-fat habit. Some children who cannot or will not drink milk will eat yogurt, cheese, or ice milk.

Children who eat breakfast perform better in school, especially if they eat the right kind of breakfast. Although most people do not feed their children cookies and soft drinks for breakfast, some of the foods marketed as cereal or health bars are hardly different—the main ingredient is sugar. Whole-grain breads and cereals with fresh fruit and not coated over with sugar make an excellent breakfast. The fiber provides a satisfied feeling that persists much longer than the quick energy swings that result from simple sugars.

Many children don't like vegetables. Parents may be able to sneak vegetables into breads, sauces, and soups and make them acceptable. There are many different ways to prepare and combine healthy fruits and vegetables. Sometimes it is best to disguise them. An opposite tack is to have the children help to prepare them, since the pride of creation may lead them to taste them as well.

Children should know that their parents think nutrition is important. Good nutrition should be learned by word, by example, and by what is available in the house to eat. Prevention of osteoporosis as well as heart disease, vascular disease, and many other adult health problems begins in childhood.

THE ELDERLY Many elderly people do not eat enough to obtain adequate nutrition. There are several reasons that make this understandable, but none to which there are no answers.

Mechanical problems with eating increase with age. Poor teeth, arthritis in the temperomandibular joint (where the jaw meets the skull), and drying of the mouth due to inadequate saliva all occur more frequently among the aged. Denture fit changes with age, especially in people with osteoporosis, so that many people need, but do not obtain, new dentures to replace ones that no longer fit properly. Drying of saliva may be a natural consequence of aging, but may also be a side effect of drugs used for depression, high blood pressure, and other medical problems.

Taste buds may become less sensitive with age. For food to be appetizing, therefore, it may need to be more flavorful. The tendency to make soft and moist foods bland may be one reason food does not seem good to many older people.

Loss of appetite is a common symptom of depression, which

is a common problem among older people. Loss of loved ones, job, income, and physical vigor can lead to depression. Depression is also a frequent side effect of some drugs used to control blood pressure and anxiety.

Many drugs taken by elderly people cause decreased appetite. Digitalis, anticoagulants, reserpine, hydralazine, aminophylline, and anti-inflammatory drugs are common causes of lost appetite among older people. Chemotherapy and radiation treatments for cancer also suppress appetite.

Access to nutritious food is a problem for many older people. If it is hard to get to the grocery store, they may rely on canned or packaged foods, which are not as nutritious as fresh foods. Milk may be hard to transport.

There are many solutions to the nutrition problems of the elderly. They should seek medical consultation with the specific question of whether any medicines might be part of the problem and whether alternative prescriptions are available. They should seek consultation with a dentist regarding mechanical problems with teeth, jaw, or saliva. They should find a grocer who will deliver milk and fresh fruits and vegetables.

Many older people live alone. Buying and cooking in single portions may be difficult. Elderly people should seek out the good nutrition and companionship of senior citizens' center meal programs or such services as Meals on Wheels. Careful meal planning, special provisions for freezing and storing leftovers, and imaginative use of extra foods such as in soups are helpful as well. Good books on nutrition and food planning for the elderly are available in bookstores and libraries.

Some studies of older people, particularly those in nursing homes, suggest that vitamin deficiencies are more common among older people. Inadequate food intake may not be the only reason. Older people may not absorb certain vitamins as well as younger people. Anemia and mental disorders can result from vitamin deficiency, but should be regarded as such only if consultation with a physician leads to confirmatory tests. Vitamin and mineral supplements to maintain RDAs make sense for older people, but using vitamins to self-treat specific symptoms without a confirmed diagnosis does not.

THE POOR   Poor people, who need good and inexpensive food, may be duped into buying the least nutrition for the most money if they do not understand what constitutes good nutrition. Many poor people live on diets of candy bars and soft drinks. The nutritional value of such foods is almost zero, so the cost in dollars per unit of nutrition is very high. The hunger satisfaction of such foods is so short-lived that they are not even valuable for that.

Potatoes, whole-grain breads and cereals, and skim milk are the best nutritional bargains. Soybeans, beans, and rice are adequate and less-expensive sources of protein than meat—red meat has too much fat and is too expensive. The less-expensive forms of red meat, like hamburger and hot dogs, are cheaper because they have too much fat in them. Chicken and fish are the least expensive and most healthful meats.

THE RICH   The diets of many rich people are even more deficient and harmful than those of poor people. A well-marbled steak, a thick slice of prime rib, or a lobster basted in butter are symbols of affluence; they are also loaded with cholesterol. Those who can afford fine wines and other alcoholic beverages may keep their stomachs irritated with alcohol and soothed with antacids, resulting in calcium deprivation. Milk, baked potatoes, and bran cereal are among the healthiest of foods, but they are hardly staples of the gourmet diet.

Life in the fast lane is seldom conducive to good nutrition since home-grown and home-cooked foods are often replaced by airline foods and heavily sauced restaurant fare. Many people who live that life-style eat little or nothing for breakfast and lunch and then consume large amounts of poorly balanced foods late at night.

VEGETARIANS   Vegetarian diets are usually low in fat and high in fiber and bulk. Those aspects of the vegetarian diet are good, except that the high-bulk aspect of the diet means that more calcium and other minerals will be lost in the stool. Vegetarians also have more estrogen in their stools, so estrogen depletion could be slightly aggravated by high-bulk, vegetarian diets.

Vegetarians who do not drink milk have particular difficulty absorbing enough calcium. They should take calcium pills. Since many foods are forbidden on a vegetarian diet, vegetarians must be more careful that they consume all essential nutrients. The key to a healthful vegetarian diet is consumption of a great variety of foods, including fortified foods, such as fortified soy milk.

THE OVERWEIGHT   "Overweight" is a relative term. If we consider only bone health, we would not think of many people as being overweight. If you are so overweight that you cannot exercise properly, that would interfere with bone health. However, there is generally a positive correlation between weight and bone strength—that is, people who are overweight have stronger bones. Fat people are less likely to have osteoporosis than thin people.

However, the advantage of being overweight just about ends with the statistical hedge against osteoporosis. A study in 1983 showed that people who were 10–20 percent overweight may have longer lives than people who were underweight. In that study, the ideal weight was considered as that which the insurance industry had accepted as being most healthful based upon 1959 statistics. The study showed that underweight and very overweight people died earlier than those who were slightly overweight. Slightly overweight, by those standards, is still fairly thin. The average American is twenty-five pounds overweight, by those standards, so anyone above average begins to get into the higher mortality range. The "50-50-50" rule is still regarded as nearly correct—anyone over fifty who is fifty pounds or more overweight has his life expectancy reduced by 50 percent.

People who are overweight can diet without harming their

bones or general health: they need to follow all the recommendations for a healthy diet, but they must consume fewer calories. Diets that exclude groups of foods, allow excesses of certain foods, and otherwise make extreme changes in the balance of what you eat are likely to be harmful to your bones and general health. Furthermore, such diets are not likely to have any lasting effect on your weight.

If you need to lose weight, the surest course is to follow the undramatic but sound and sensible reducing diet recommendations of such programs as Weight Watchers, TOPS, Diet Center, and others that encourage low-calorie, balanced diets and lead to a permanent change in eating habits. Books such as *Jane Brody's Nutrition Book* give the same sort of solid advice. Do not fall for fad and gimmick diets. Anyone can call himself or herself a "nutritionist" or "health food expert." If you need personal guidance about your diet, ask your physician to help you find a reputable dietitian, seek a dietitian who displays the initials "R.D." (registered dietitian), or choose someone with an established community reputation for sound diet advice.

THE UNDERWEIGHT   Extreme avoidance of food and pathologic weight reduction is called anorexia nervosa. Anorexia nervosa was once thought to be a disease of young women; there have been well-known, tragic examples of deaths of young women from anorexia nervosa. However, anorexia nervosa has recently been occurring more frequently among men and among older people.

Such extreme nutritional deprivation causes disastrous effects to all aspects of health, including bone health. People with anorexia nervosa think they are fat when by all reasonable standards they are not. It is very important to recognize the problem early and seek the help of professionals who understand how to treat this disease. If a reducing diet has so captured your imagination that the weight reduction goes on beyond the original goal, seek help.

SUMMARY OF HEALTHFUL DIET PRACTICES

Drink plenty of skim milk or eat nonfat yogurt. Eat boiled or baked potatoes with their skins, and whole-grain breads and cereals. Eat fresh green and yellow vegetables and fruits; if fresh is not available, fresh-frozen is better than canned. Avoid butter, whole milk, cream, bacon, animal fats, shellfish, fatty meats, and sugar. Lean meats, especially fish and chicken, broiled or baked without grease are good. Make soup from leftovers of fresh foods; leach calcium from soupbones with vinegar. Do not add salt to food. If you must carefully limit your salt because of high blood pressure or fluid retention, buy low-sodium milk. Take only enough vitamin and mineral supplements to ensure that you get your RDA. It is unwise to take supplements much in excess of the RDA, except when extra calcium and/or fluoride are needed, as described in the next chapter.

7

Calcium and Fluoride

IF YOU can get the essential nutrients from what you eat, without eating things that are bad for you, it is best not to take pills. Unfortunately, many people cannot manage their diets that well. They may need certain nutrients in such high doses that they find it impractical to consume them in food.

A multivitamin pill that ensures you get your recommended daily allowance of all vitamins is the most universally accepted diet supplement. Many people need to take calcium pills to protect their bones. We do not know enough about fluoride pills to make a general statement about how many people might need them, but the evidence that fluoride supplements may help is strong enough to warrant detailed consideration of what we do know.

VITAMINS

Vitamins were defined and discussed in the previous chapter. The subject is included again here, without details, because you should consider vitamins and minerals when you shop for diet supplements.

There has been so much research and so much experience with vitamin supplements that it is safe to assume that a vitamin pill or capsule that provides you with your RDA of all essential vitamins is safe. The same assurance cannot be given about vitamin excesses. We do not know all the long-term effects of extraordinarily high vitamin intake. In 1984 in the United States, thirty-eight infant deaths were attributed to a vitamin-E supplement everyone considered harmless. The FDA requires that vitamins be 98 percent pure and that the other 2 percent of the ingredients be harmless in recommended doses. No one is sure what may happen if that 2 percent is multiplied by doses that greatly exceed the recommended ones. There are delicate balances between the thousands of substances in our bodies, and we do not know which ones we upset if we overload ourselves with some particular vitamin or mineral.

Unless your diet provides you with all the vitamins you need, take a supplement that ensures the recommended daily allowance. If you get a little extra because of your diet, that will not hurt—but do not take excesses of vitamin supplements. Even if you accept those recommendations, though, you are still faced with some confusing choices because there are literally hundreds of vitamin and mineral supplements on the market.

If you know that your diet is deficient in only one or two vitamins or minerals, or that you have some special need for extra of a particular one, it may be best for you to select a supplement that specifically applies to your need. Calcium is the best example of such a specific need, as will be discussed a bit later. Otherwise, it is usually simplest and most economical to take one pill or capsule to provide you with all the supplements you might need.

Most multivitamins should supply you with your RDA of vitamins A, B_1, B_2, B_6, B_{12}, C, D, E, niacin, copper, manganese, magnesium, iodine, and zinc. If you are getting D from fortified milk or with a calcium supplement, you may not need it in your multivitamin. Iron, contained in many multivitamins, is more important to some people than others—women who have menstrual periods, for example. Folic acid, pantothenic acid, biotin, and others of the trace minerals are also present in many multi-vitamins.

There is a huge variety in the composition, availability, and price of multivitamins. You need to study the labels and perhaps enlist the help of your pharmacist when you decide what you and your family should take—and how much you are going to have to pay. You should not pay for excesses or gimmicks such as "natural" vitamins. Your best bet is to buy laboratory-prepared, clearly labeled pills or capsules from a place you trust. Prices vary, so compare different brands of the same thing. Once you decide what is best, you can probably save a great deal of money if you buy in large quantity. When you compare, you need to find out what is available in large quantities and what the markdowns are.

Most vitamin and mineral supplements are called "multivitamins." Some labeling is just by brand name and does not make that designation. Read the fine print on the ingredients labels to know what you are getting. That is not always easy, even if you have exceptionally good eyesight.

Some labels will say that "2 pills provide . . . ," or "1 pill 3 times a day provides . . . ," or "so many ounces provide . . . ," then follow with a list of ingredients and amounts, leaving you with the task of figuring out how much is in each pill so you can compare it to another brand. If you overlook that qualifier of how the amounts are supplied, you can misinterpret what you are getting by 100 percent or more. Doses may be listed in grams, milligrams, micrograms, or units. Even more confusing, the weight may refer to the whole molecule or just the active portion. Adequately labeled supplements should simplify some of this for you by listing the percentage of the RDA, so you do not have to worry about units of weight.

Some multivitamins are designed and marketed to provide for the needs of special groups. Often the "special" nature of the vitamins consists only of advertising and marketing devices, and the vitamins contain extra amounts of some ingredients that few people need. An exception that is worthy of attention is the prenatal vitamins marketed for pregnant women. Prenatal vitamins usually contain extra calcium. If you are going to take multivitamins and calcium supplements, it is worth comparing labels and prices to see if prenatal vitamins would have any advantage for you. Since some multivitamins contain calcium supplements and some calcium supplements contain vitamins, you need not pay extra just because the label says "prenatal"—but do include the prenatals in your comparisons.

If you are worried about osteoporosis, calcium is the supplement of greatest concern. Unfortunately, wise shopping for calcium supplements is difficult. The problems don't end with the great number of available prenatal vitamins, multivitamins with calcium, calcium supplements with vitamins, and plain calcium supplements. Label information about calcium is confusing at best and sometimes all but incomprehensible. Sometimes you should check a product off your list of possibilities simply because you cannot understand the label. Most often, however, you can interpret the labels if you know some of the tricks.

CALCIUM

As you learned in the last chapter, some people need almost twice as much calcium as others and almost twice as much calcium as the recommended daily allowance. People who drink a great deal of milk or eat many dairy products may get all the calcium they need, but most other people do not. In the case of calcium, there are often reasons to exceed the RDA. The reasons are that the RDA for calcium is not the same for everyone, and there are a very large number of people who have a need that exceeds the ordinary. In light of present knowledge, the current RDA is probably set too low to cover the needs of most of the population.

In the discussion of vitamins, I presented good reasons to avoid excesses. Even those people who have the greatest need to exceed the RDA for calcium should take no more than twice the recommended allowance. Huge excesses of calcium are useless and possibly dangerous.

Calcium-rich diets and calcium supplements that provide a total of 1,500 mg of calcium per day do not cause any problems for the majority of people. High levels of calcium in the blood are very dangerous, but the body works very efficiently to keep blood calcium within a safe range, regardless of calcium intake. If you have some disease that interferes with calcium balance, you need your physician's advice about how much or how little calcium to take.

Kidney stones can occur because of abnormal calcium balance. They are fairly common, very painful, and sometimes health-threatening. Some—but not all—kidney stones contain calcium phosphate or calcium oxalate. If you ever pass a kidney stone you should save it and have it analyzed. If it contains no calcium, you have less reason to worry about absorbing too much calcium.

If you have kidney stones that do contain calcium, you may or may not have some reason to restrict your calcium intake. Many people who form calcium stones have something wrong with their calcium-balance mechanism, often with their parathyroid hormones. If the balance can be restored, there is less reason to worry about calcium excess. Some people form calcium stones in combination with uric acid stones, a problem that can be corrected by taking uric acid medication (allopurinol). Some people form calcium oxalate stones because they absorb too much oxalate, not because they absorb too much calcium. However, some people do absorb too much calcium.

If you have had kidney stones, there is reason to be concerned about taking extra calcium. Drink a great deal of water to avoid dehydration. Thiazide diuretic medicines reduce calcium excretion by the kidney and, thereby, may conserve calcium while reducing the risk of calcium stones. However, do not decide to reduce your calcium intake unless such a reduction is required because you form stones. If you can correct the tendency to form stones some other way, you should not deprive yourself of the calcium your bones need. People who truly absorb too much calcium will not suffer in their bones from reduced calcium in their diets, but people who form stones for any other reason will suffer in their bones if their calcium intake is too low.

You may have been told you have calcium deposits in or around a joint. The shoulder, in the tendons near the joint, is a common place for such deposits. Calcium deposits do not occur because of too much calcium in the diet. Do not reduce your consumption of calcium because of a deposit in or around a joint. The same is true with bone spurs and other overgrowths of bone. Bone thickens at points of stress, sometimes forming projections of bone called osteophytes, or spurs. Bony overgrowths have nothing to do with excess calcium. You should not consider bone spurs or calcium deposits when you decide how much calcium you need in your diet.

Certain heart conditions are treated with drugs called "calcium blockers" or "channel blockers." Calcium in food and calcium supplements do not interfere with the action of these drugs. Do not be afraid to consume calcium because you are taking a calcium-blocker drug.

Calcium is abundant in nature. The calcium ion has a positive charge, which attracts a negative ion. The calcium in many plants is linked to oxalate or phytate ions. Calcium oxalate and calcium phytate do not dissolve well in the human intestine, and in spite of high-calcium contents, foods rich in these substances (e.g., whole grains, spinach, asparagus) do not provide your bones with much calcium.

Many multivitamin-mineral preparations contain some calcium. If you read the labels carefully, you will find that the amount of calcium in such multiple preparations, except for the prenatals, is so small that you can just about ignore it. One reason is the size of the pill. The molecules that contain calcium are large molecules, and the requirements for calcium are substantial. If there is anywhere near the amount of calcium you need in a pill, there will be little room for much else.

As I have said, calcium in nature is often linked to some form of phosphate. Calcium phosphates do not dissolve well in the intestines. The phosphates dissolve only partially, and some of the calcium is absorbed. The amount absorbed depends upon individual characteristics and the contents of your intestines at the time. Commercial preparations of calcium phosphate supplements contain about 29 percent calcium. Whether the extra phosphorus helps or hurts is controversial and probably depends upon what other phosphates are present in your diet. Too much phosphate is likely to interfere with calcium absorption.

If you go to the store to buy calcium, you will find that it is combined with either phosphate or with a form of organic acid. Organic acids are molecules containing carbon, oxygen, and hydrogen. One hydrogen atom becomes free in solution, leaving the rest of the molecule with a negative charge, which attracts positively charged ions such as calcium. The combination of an organic-acid ion and a positive ion is called an organic salt. Most calcium supplements in the stores are organic salts. Unless you have studied chemistry, this terminology is unfamiliar, but it will help you with some of the less well understood, but much more familiar, words you find on labels.

The smallest organic acid is carbonic acid. Carbonic acid has just one carbon atom. The salts of carbonic acid are called carbonates. Calcium carbonate is the most widely sold form of calcium supplement. Calcium from oyster shells is mostly calcium carbonate.

Because the carbonate ion is small, as organic acid ions go, the calcium takes up a relatively large part of each molecule—about 40 percent. This is where label interpretation gets tricky. If the label says each pill contains 500 mg of calcium carbonate, you can figure you are getting 40 percent of that, or 200 mg, of calcium in each pill. However, if the label says each pill contains 500 mg of calcium as calcium carbonate, then you are getting 500 mg of calcium in each pill. Quite a difference. If the wording on the label is so obscure that you cannot tell what it means, select a different brand.

Remember to be careful that the label information pertains to what is in one pill. Many calcium pill labels will say that the recommended dose schedule is so many pills per day and that if you take that many pills each day you will get so much calcium. That leaves you to figure out how much calcium you are getting in each pill, find out the price for various quantities of that form of calcium, and determine what is your best bargain in terms of milligrams of actual calcium per penny. A calculator is a handy tool when you shop for calcium, because the situation becomes a little more complicated—calcium carbonate is not the only calcium salt sold for calcium supplements.

Calcium supplements are also available as calcium lactate, calcium gluconate, and calcium ascorbate. Some supplements contain various combinations of these calcium salts, plus calcium carbonate or phosphate.

Calcium lactate is the salt of calcium and lactic acid. Lactate contains three carbon atoms, so it is larger than carbonate. Therefore, calcium makes up a smaller percentage of each molecule. Commercial preparations contain about 13 percent calcium. One 600-mg pill of calcium lactate contains only about 78 mg of calcium. The name lactate may have some appeal because it sounds like lactose, the sugar in milk. Lactose aids calcium absorption. However, lactose is a double sugar combination of glucose and galactose, containing fourteen carbon atoms. Lactate is not a form of lactose.

Calcium gluconate is the calcium salt of gluconic acid. As you might imagine, gluconic acid is very similar to the simple sugar glucose—both contain six carbon atoms. The noncalcium portion of calcium gluconate takes up even more of the molecule than calcium lactate. Only about 9 percent of a calcium gluconate pill is calcium. To obtain 1,000 mg of calcium as calcium gluconate, you might have to take more than twenty tablets of the 500-mg size. Calcium gluconate is very sweet and may irritate your stomach.

Ascorbic acid, another name for vitamin C, is also an organic acid. Ascorbic acid can form a salt with calcium. Some calcium supplements contain calcium ascorbate, and some vitamin-C supplements are calcium ascorbate. The problem with calcium ascorbate as a calcium supplement is that ascorbate, like gluconate, is a six-carbon molecule, so only a small percentage of the pill is calcium.

Both calcium gluconate and calcium lactate dissolve easily. You can be sure that you will absorb most of the calcium from calcium gluconate and calcium lactate, but they are generally more expensive and less convenient than calcium carbonate. For most people, calcium carbonate is the best supplement. All calcium pills are big and hard to swallow. Many are scored so you can cut them in two if you have trouble swallowing whole ones, but then you have to swallow twice as many. Calcium carbonate is chalky but the taste is not terrible. Chewable, flavored calcium carbonate is available both as a calcium supplement and, in lower dosage, as an antacid.

Calcium carbonate dissolves in stomach acid. People who have no stomach acid (a condition that can occur postsurgery, or from gastric cancer, chronic gastritis, or other, less common conditions) or who have neutralized their stomach acid with medication will not absorb calcium carbonate well. If you have no stomach acid, you should take calcium gluconate or lactate.

Some people who take high doses of calcium carbonate become constipated. If exercise, bulk diet, fruit juices, and high fluid intake do not solve the problem, it may be necessary to modify the calcium regimen. Calcium lactate or calcium gluconate may be less constipating. A more determined effort to obtain adequate calcium from diet rather than from pills may be wise. Sometimes overzealous supplementation leads to excess calcium: remember that there is no advantage, except when pregnant or nursing, to ingest more than a total (from diet and pills) of 1,500 mg of calcium daily and that overdoses may be constipating.

Many calcium supplements contain vitamin D. If you need a vitamin-D supplement, are not drinking any fortified milk, and are not getting vitamin D from a multivitamin, you might find such a combination of calcium and vitamin D to be the best value. You don't have to take calcium and vitamin D in the same pill; do so only if you need the vitamin D and that proves to be the most convenient and economical way to get it. Check the labels carefully, because some brand-name calcium supplements contain vitamin D in their smaller pills but not in their larger pills of similar name.

Remember that a cup of fortified milk will give you 100 units of vitamin D (one-fourth of the RDA for children and half the RDA for adults) and almost 300 mg of calcium. If you drink milk with your meals, you will not need to take much calcium and vitamin D. If you take calcium carbonate, it is best to take it with water on an empty stomach so that your stomach acids dissolve the pills. You may need both milk and calcium, but you absorb more calcium if you do not take them together. Milk neutralizes some of the stomach acid, and taking in large quantities of calcium at once is less efficient than spacing it in smaller doses.

It may sound like a great deal of trouble to figure out how much and what kind of calcium you need and what your best buy is. It is worth taking the time to go through that once, because you can then buy large quantities and stop thinking about it. You need to include a calcium supplement as part of your daily routine for life. Think of it more as food than as medicine.

FLUORIDE

Fluoride is the negatively charged ion of the element fluorine, which in its pure form exists as a gas. Fluoride ions are present in small quantities throughout nature. They are often linked to the positive ion of sodium, forming the relatively simple compound sodium fluoride.

In Denmark, in 1932, Dr. P. Flemming Moller, a roentgenologist, and Dr. Sk. V. Gudjohnsson, an industrial health physician, described an affliction of workers who had been exposed to cryolite dust. Cryolite is a mineral principally composed of sodium fluoride and aluminum fluoride. The workers suffered from vomiting, nausea, and anemia, and their bones appeared very dense in X rays. The Danish doctors proved that the workers were ill from fluoride poisoning. They even suggested that the fluorides, in lower doses, might be beneficial for such diseases as osteoporosis. In 1944, Fuller Albright, the pioneer in the care of osteoporosis whose more substantial contributions are discussed in Chapter 5, considered fluoride as a treatment for osteoporosis. Albright tried giving sodium fluoride to osteoporosis patients but found that it did not help.

Nothing further about fluoride treatment for osteoporosis appeared in the medical literature until 1961. In 1954 a report to the American Association for the Advancement of Science stated that people who lived in areas where the water was rich in fluoride seemed to have less osteoporosis. In the 1960s and early 1970s researchers began to explore more thoroughly the idea of using fluoride to treat osteoporosis. Early reports about effectiveness were not convincing, and there were worries that in some instances fluorides seemed to make things worse. Fluoride treatment had the reputation of making the X rays look better but making the bones weaker.

In spite of problems with clinical safety and effectiveness, physicians and research chemists of the past two decades have been less willing to abandon the idea of using fluorides for osteoporosis than they were in the 1940s and 1950s. Osteoporosis has become a bigger problem, and the other attempts at cure have not been totally successful. In addition, there were some encouraging clinical responses, and there was some information from scientific experiments that stimulated researchers to keep trying to find a use for fluorides.

Fluoride ions are found on the surfaces of the hydroxyapatite crystals in bone; fluorides are also found deeply embedded within the crystals. Apatite crystals that contain fluoride are less soluble and more resistant to resorption than crystals without fluoride. Fluoride ions are also found to be active in the energy-producing chemistry of cells, including bone-forming cells.

Bone production seems to be stimulated by the presence of fluorides. When fluoride ions are present in abundance, the activity of the bone-forming osteoblasts increases. The osteoblasts lay down thicker seams of new bone. As a result, fluoride-treated bone is less porous than untreated bone.

Since 1970, several centers treating patients with severe osteoporosis with high doses of fluoride have reported favorable results. Pain from spinal fractures has diminished more rapidly in patients who take fluoride. The urine of patients who take fluoride contains less calcium, possibly indicative that the bones are retaining calcium better. The bones appear more dense on X rays, densitometry, and Compton-scatter studies. And, most important, the incidence of broken bones decreases in and after the second year of treatment.

So there is real hope that fluorides may provide all those benefits. Unfortunately, not all reports are as favorable and there are some real uncertainties.

Some of the initial negativism about fluorides was due to the fact that fluorides can make bone brittle. Chalk is dense but breaks easily, and so, in some circumstances, do fluoride-treated bones. If fluoride doses are too high, if the kidneys do not adequately clear excess fluoride, or if there is not enough calcium available to keep the new bone crystals calcium-rich, brittle bone can result from fluoride treatment.

At this point, we are just discovering what the correct dose of fluoride should be. We are aware that some doses seem to have been successful, but there is much left to learn. We don't know how long patients should keep taking fluorides. The safe "window," the range between being ineffective and being dangerous, is more narrow for fluorides than for many naturally occurring substances. The 1980 recommendations of the National Academy of Sciences and the National Research Council were that fluoride should be consumed in daily doses of 1.5–4 mg. Fluoride is considered definitely toxic at 1,000 mg and lethal between 2,000 and 20,000 mg. The doses used to treat severe osteoporosis have been in the range of 45–150 mg of sodium fluoride per day. It takes 2.2 mg of sodium fluoride to supply 1 mg of fluoride, so 45 mg of sodium fluoride is actually about 20 mg of fluoride.

Fluoride is normally present in blood in the range of 0.15–0.25 part per million, a very small but measurable amount. With safe and effective treatment the blood levels increase to 0.25–0.50 ppm. We do not know if it is necessary or even meaningful to monitor blood levels during treatment.

In addition to experiencing uncertainty about safe and effective dosage, many patients experience side effects from fluoride treatment. Stomach and intestinal irritation is the most common. Some people avoid stomach irritation if they begin with low doses and increase their fluoride intake gradually. The gastrointestinal side effects can usually be treated so that fluoride treatment can continue, but the side effects should not be treated with aluminum-containing antacids, since they interfere with calcium absorption and it is particularly important that patients who are taking fluorides keep their calcium up. Another common side effect of fluorides is joint pain and arthritis-like symptoms. These are usually transient and controlled without abandoning the fluoride treatment.

About one-third of patients who take fluorides do not seem to get the benefits that the other two-thirds do. We know that people who are calcium-deficient or who have osteomalacia may form bone of poor quality if they take fluorides before they correct the calcium deficiency, but that is probably not a full explanation. Among the challenges to researchers are ways to identify who will and who will not respond to fluoride and ways to explain the differences between those groups.

Although thousands of patients have been observed over several years of fluoride treatments, not enough time has elapsed to be sure about unrecognized ill effects. There has been concern over vision loss because it occurred in two patients, but whether or not fluoride was the immediate cause was doubtful. Microscopic changes in the thyroid glands and kidneys occur in animals given high doses of fluoride, but thyroid and kidney dysfunction does not seem to occur in humans who undergo fluoride treatments.

Doctors can be slow to recognize complications of new treatments. When the treatments extend over a long time and the patients develop other illnesses and take other medicines, drug effects that appear months or years after treatment begins may be hard to recognize.

With all this conflict and uncertainty, how does one decide about taking fluorides? The one unarguable answer is that one should not experiment with self-care by taking large doses of fluorides: there is too much danger and too much uncertainty. If you are going to take fluorides in anywhere near the doses suggested for the treatment of osteoporosis, do it with the advice and supervision of a physician who is familiar with fluoride treatments.

If you think fluoride treatment may be indicated for you or a loved one, seek your doctor's advice. If your physician does not know about fluorides, ask for a referral to a physician who does. Even after you talk to a physician about fluorides, you may not be satisfied. The medical community is not uniform in its attitude about fluoride treatments. Some physicians strongly endorse fluoride treatment and work through the problems to provide it to their patients; other physicians regard fluoride treatment as too new and uncertain, and will not prescribe it.

If your physician recommends fluoride treatment, there are

still problems with obtaining it. Your physician will guide you to the best answer, but it may not be a very good one. The problem is that there are no convenient dose forms of fluoride that are commercially available for the treatment of osteoporosis. The reasons for this involve the law and government agency control over untested drugs. As of 1984, the FDA stated that the use of sodium fluoride for the treatment of osteoporosis was still considered experimental and was not generally recognized by the scientific and medical community as safe and effective for that purpose. The stance of the FDA limits the availability of sodium fluoride products.

Fluoride has been recognized as safe and effective in the prevention of tooth decay. The effective dose for prevention of tooth decay is quite small compared to that for osteoporosis. Sodium fluoride pills of 2.2 mg (1 mg of fluoride) are stocked by most pharmacies. Physicians who are convinced of the wisdom of giving high doses of fluoride to their osteoporosis patients may legally prescribe large quantities of these pills. However, this is very inconvenient for the patients, since commonly prescribed doses might require that the patient take thirty sodium fluoride pills per day—not to mention all the calcium pills that are needed.

One American manufacturer (Mericon) makes a capsule containing 8 mg of sodium fluoride, which is somewhat more convenient than the 2.2-mg tablets. The capsule also contains calcium. Putting calcium in the same capsule with fluoride sounds like a good idea, but it may not be. Calcium and fluoride mixed may form calcium fluoride, which is relatively insoluble, so neither drug may be absorbed as well as if taken separately.

Sodium fluoride is easy to manufacture. It can be mixed with orange juice or poured into capsules. Some physicians have supplied their patients with sodium fluoride in those ways, but that is cumbersome for both patient and physician. Sodium fluoride is also made in controlled-release capsules in a convenient dose form, but few physicians can prescribe them and few patients can buy them. The manufacturer complies with the FDA recommendations that use of sodium fluoride in the doses needed for osteoporosis be restricted. The physician must apply for and receive an investigational new drug (IND) permit before prescribing such capsules. Investigational new drug numbers are not simply awarded to physicians in good standing: the physician who requests an IND number must demonstrate knowledge of the drug and outline the way in which he or she plans to use it for treatment and research. The physician must agree to comply with regulations for the investigation and reporting of drug effects, which are beyond the scope of most doctors' practices.

The FDA is not simply being obstructionist. The agency's stance is to protect the public from the widespread use of a treatment method that has not been thoroughly investigated.

The National Institutes of Health encouraged a double-blind, randomized clinical trial of fluoride treatment of osteoporosis currently being conducted under the sponsorship of the National Institute of Arthritis, Metabolism, and Digestive Diseases. Studies are being done at the Mayo Clinic in Rochester, Minnesota, and at Henry Ford Hospital in Detroit. The studies began as early as 1968, but conclusions upon which the FDA could base a decision are not expected until the late 1980s. One of the teams conducting the NIH-endorsed trial issued an interim report in the February 25, 1982, issue of the *New England Journal of Medicine.* The study compared the occurrence rates of spinal fractures in women who were being treated in various ways. They found that those who were treated with a combination of calcium, estrogens, and fluorides did the best.

The 1982 interim report and studies from Israel and elsewhere have strongly encouraged those who believe in the benefits of flourides and have increased pressures to make fluorides more readily available. The FDA, however, will await more complete and conclusive reports. Meanwhile, patients who take fluorides must take the 2.2-mg tablets, the Mericon capsules of fluoride and calcium (Florical), powders or capsules prepared under the direction of their physician, or capsules prescribed by a physician with an IND number.

As of 1984, there is still much we do not know about fluorides. We do not know the ideal dose or the ideal length of time to take the drug. We do not know if there might be a better compound than the commonly used sodium fluoride. We are not certain we know all the complications. We do not know why some patients don't respond to fluoride, or how to select the patients who will respond. We are not certain if low doses of fluoride help to prevent osteoporosis or would provide satisfactory treatment for mild cases of osteoporosis. We do not know what tests are best to monitor the safety and effectiveness of fluoride treatment.

In spite of all those unknowns, it has seemed to me, in my practice, that there are some patients who should be treated with fluorides. Many conservative physicians agree with me. It is a matter of weighing risks and benefits. People who have the severely painful and disfiguring problem of repeated spinal fractures need treatment to restore lost bone strength. Calcium and estrogens preserve bone strength, but they do not restore it well. Although exercise restores bone strength, it takes a long time to do so, and for many patients who are weak and in pain, exercise is not a practical short-term solution. Fluorides do not always work and sometimes cause trouble, but in desperate situations it is worth taking some chances.

Whether patients who have had broken hips and wrists, or who have evidence of osteoporosis but no fractures, should take fluorides is more doubtful under present circumstances. As we understand fluorides better and become more skilled in using them, I suspect physicians and patients will be more willing to use them under some less-than-desperate circumstances.

If you take fluorides, take them only under a doctor's prescription and continue under the doctor's care throughout the time you take them. Most physicians prescribe 40–80 mg of sodium fluoride per day (about 20–35 mg of fluoride). If your kidneys do not function normally, you may need a lower dose and closer-than-usual scrutiny. Most treatment courses run two to three years; some physicians recommend even longer treatment. Do not be discouraged if you develop new fractures during the first year: building bone takes time. The important decrease in fracture rate among people who are helped by fluorides comes *after* the first year of treatment.

If you are going to take fluorides, do not look upon them as a simple answer to a complicated problem. No one recommends fluorides as the only treatment for osteoporosis. Fluorides, when they are used, must be used in conjunction with a balanced program of good nutrition, calcium supplementation, exercise, and often hormones. Without a balanced and complete program, fluorides may produce bone of poor quality and defeat the intended purpose. It is often best to begin a balanced program before you start with fluorides so that you are ready to make good bone when the fluorides trip the bone-making switch.

8

Fractures: Where, How, and Why?

BREAKS IN BONES are called fractures. Fracture is the proper term whether the bone is broken apart or just cracked, whether it is broken all the way through or just on one surface, whether it is broken into two pieces or many, and whether or not the broken edge comes through the skin. The question "Is it fractured or broken?" has no meaning—there is no difference.

Bones fracture in different ways. The shape and strength of the bone and the characteristics of the injury determine the particular way the bone breaks. Short, stout, biscuit-shaped bones, like the vertebral bodies, break in different ways from long, cylindrical bones, like the femur (thighbone).

Every movement you make causes stress to your bones. Your muscles and gravity both pull on your bones; this creates stresses that can break them. Bones don't break from every stress, since they have internal strength and the muscles protect them. If the stress exceeds the internal strength of the bone and your ability to counteract the stress with your muscles, the bone will break. Sometimes nothing more than unbalanced muscle pull and gravity causes a fracture; at other times, some outside force adds the stress that leads to a break.

Some weight and muscle forces are directed straight in line with the main axis of the bone, so that little twisting and bending force is present. A force may act straight along the axis of the bone either to push it together in upon itself (axial compression) or to pull it directly apart (distraction). Bones are very strong in their resistance to fracture from such pure axial load forces.

Pure distraction forces are rather uncommon. Few bones are pulled directly apart. One example is the seat-belt fracture. If an accident victim is thrust up and forward at high speed, and at the same time held down by a seat belt, the forces may be great enough to tear a vertebra by pulling it apart—a bad injury but usually not as bad as the head injury that might have occurred had those forces not been contained by the seat belt. Except for such very violent injuries, pure distraction forces are uncommon, and even osteoporotic bones are resistant to being pulled directly apart.

Gravity is forever trying to pull us toward the center of the earth. Sometimes it does so very abruptly, as when we slip from our feet or fall from a ladder. Compression forces are, therefore, very common. Just by standing upright, you place considerable compression force through the long axis of your spine. Sometimes pure compression forces break bones, but more often fractures are caused by compression in combination with other forces.

If you place a paper cup on a flat surface and try to crush it by placing an even force down around the whole top, you will feel the resistance to fracture of a hollow, tubular structure loaded by pure axial compression. Of course, a paper cup is very weak and you can overcome that resistance, but you can appreciate how much more resistance the cup has to axial compression loads than it has when you bend it from one side. If you do the same experiment with an aluminum can, you will sense similar behavior in a structure with more internal strength. If you repeat the experiment with a plain straight drinking glass, you observe the difference in a material that has tremendous resistance to fracture from direct load but a tendency to fly apart in many pieces if struck from the side. None of these materials are exactly like bone, but you can apply the physical principles you observe to what you know about bone.

Pure compression, straight along the axis of the whole bone, seldom occurs in long bones. Long bones curve, so that the forces of compression travel along one or the other side of the bone. The action is more like what you think of as a bending force than a compression force.

The short, cube-shaped bones of the front of the spine (vertebral bodies) absorb forces that are more nearly pure compression forces than do the long bones. The vertebral bodies are not physically separated from the arches of bone to the sides and back of the spine, but the forces that act upon the bodies are different. The vertebral bodies may fracture while the rest of the bone of that vertebra remains intact, especially in people with osteoporosis.

The theoretical line about which your weight is balanced, the axis of your weight, is called your center of gravity. When you stand, your vertebral bodies are near your center of gravity. Therefore, the force of gravity tends to compress your vertebral bodies. The discs that cushion the top and bottom of each vertebral body spread the stresses so that some bending stresses are converted to compression stresses.

Vertebral bodies are built to withstand compression. Multiple, interconnecting beams of bone efficiently distribute stresses. Materials like the drinking glass mentioned above resist compression because of their overall geometry, but they shatter if you isolate and compress one part of them. The trabecular bone of vertebral bodies is not brittle in that way.

If the internal architecture of a vertebral body weakens, as from osteoporosis, it will not be able to withstand as much compression stress. A sudden force may cause the vertebral body to collapse down upon itself, like a biscuit would if you hit it with your fist. An accumulation of little forces could have the same end result, like a biscuit might look if you poked it with your fingertip several times. Either way, the end result is called a "compression fracture." Compression fractures are not often caused by pure compression, since forces usually are directed eccentrically along one side of the vertebral body. The center of gravity is usually a little in front of the spine; during lifting and bending efforts it may be fairly far in front, so forces are usually greater along the front (anterior) side of the vertebral body. Compression fractures are often wedged, so that the front of the vertebral body is crushed down more than the back. Wedging contributes to the bent-over, round-shouldered posture of people with spinal fractures from osteoporosis. These all-too-common injuries are sometimes called "anterior wedge compression fractures."

When you stand, the long bones of your legs carry the force of your body weight from the floor to your spine. The center of gravity of your body weight usually passes between your legs, so your weight is trying to bend your legs into a bowlegged position. When you shift your weight to one leg, your center of gravity passes close to where the forces are transmitted through your knee. Your thigh, at the hip, is almost always to the side of your center of gravity. The top of your femur, where it bends to turn in toward your hip joint, experiences much more bending stress than the bones near your knee.

Long bones are built to withstand bending stresses. Although they are hollow tubes, their walls are quite thick. The walls of the femur, in particular, are very thick. The proportion of wall to central space of the middle portion of the femur is more like a pencil than like a drinking straw. The thick wall (cortex) is composed of bone with densely packed crystals. The thickness and density of the cortex of a long bone provide strength to resist tremendous bending and twisting stresses, but they make the bone a bit brittle. If a force is great enough to overcome the tremendous internal strength of such bones, especially if that force is applied very rapidly, the bone may break into more than two pieces. A fracture that contains more than two pieces is called a "comminuted fracture."

You can break a pencil much more easily if you hold it near its ends, rather than near its middle. The farther away you apply the bending force, the less force you need to break the pencil. The same is true for bone. If you break your femur from a fall, the forces that created the stress are your weight pulling through your center of gravity, the resistance of your muscles pulling, and the resistance of whatever you strike when you fall. The further away your center of gravity, the greater the force it exerts on the bone. Since your hip is usually out to the side, further away from your center of gravity than other bones, it is the most vulnerable site.

If you bend a pencil and look at the center of it, you can see that you are pushing one side together and pulling the opposite side apart. Bending forces are combinations of compression and distraction forces. You are pulling apart—distracting—the pencil on its convex side and compressing the pencil on its concave side. When a force stresses a bone beyond its strength to resist, the bone may give way on the side of compression, the side of distraction, or both. If the bone breaks only partway through, the fracture is said to be "incomplete." Such incomplete fractures are common in the long bones of children because their bones are elastic and less brittle than those of adults. Incomplete fractures sometimes look like partially broken tree branches (thus the term "greenstick fracture"). Many compression fractures of the adult spine are also incomplete fractures.

When an adult sustains a visible fracture in the cortex of a long bone, the crack usually goes all the way through the bone— a "complete fracture." The pieces of bone do not always separate. When the broken pieces do separate, the fracture is said to be "displaced," and when they do not, it is said to be "undisplaced." Sometimes the separation of fractured pieces of bone takes the form of a bend, so that the pieces make an abnormal angle with one another, a situation in which the fracture is said to be "angulated." Two pieces of bone can be smashed in upon one another. Often, the widened end of a bone is pushed down upon the more narrow shaft of the bone, like an ice cream ball being smashed down upon the cone. Such smashed-together fractures are said to be "impacted."

Individual trabeculae, or small parts of a bone, may fracture and not show (by X ray or by direct vision) any visible sign of a break in the bone. Such fractures are called "microfractures." Microfractures that repair themselves without any symptoms or sign of their presence can be considered normal remodeling processes. If too many such fractures occur and the repair processes cannot keep up with them, symptoms and visible changes in the bone appear—a phenomenon called a "stress fracture." A bone weakened by a stress fracture may suddenly break through and displace. Many hip fractures occur from a trivial injury added to an unrecognized stress fracture.

Bones are connected at joints. Joints are sometimes, though not often, called articulations. It seems better to use one syllable rather than five or six; however, when a bone is broken into a joint, we say the fracture is an "intra-articular fracture."

Compression, distraction, and bending are not the only ways force is transmitted through bone. Falls and other stresses can also twist or apply torque to the bone. The hollow, tubular structure of bones enables them to withstand a considerable twisting stress. The forces from torque are dispersed much more efficiently by a tube than by a solid piece of the same amount and type of material.

If there is any break in the continuity of the tubular structure of a bone, stresses will not pass across that area and will accumulate around it. A weak spot in the bone may produce such a "stress riser." Anatomic bends in the bone, surgical implants with different elastic properties than the bone, holes from surgery or from tumors or infections, or anything that interferes with the smooth transmission of forces across an area can be called a stress riser. Bones are more likely to break through stress risers.

The bend in the top of the femur where it turns to the hip joint can be considered an anatomic stress riser.

If you calculate the forces your body absorbs when you fall, being careful to multiply the pounds of force by the distance from the point on the bone and adding any adverse effect from muscles pulling against the bone, you find that the forces from practically every fall exceed the strength of bone. If that is true, which it is, your bones should break every time you fall. Something else must account for the fact that they do not.

The missing factor in the calculation is the protective effect of muscles. Muscles balance the forces across the bone. Bones are almost completely covered by muscle attachments. The stresses transmitted along the bones are absorbed and dampened by muscles. People with strong, coordinated muscles can absorb great forces without breaking their bones. Falls and other injuries that occur rapidly are more likely to break bones than forces that are applied more slowly, partially because muscles can absorb more if the force is applied slowly.

If a broken piece of bone is exposed to the outside because it has torn through the skin or something has penetrated the skin in the area, the fracture is called an "open fracture." Some people call such injuries "compound fractures," but open is a simpler word, less easily confused with "comminuted," and more obviously the antonym of its opposite, the "closed fracture."

Nature tries to heal displaced fractures so the bones will end up straight. However, sometimes muscle pull angulates and displaces fractures more than nature's efforts can overcome. A physician who anticipates such an unhappy outcome may advise that the fracture be "reduced," that the pieces be put back nearer their normal positions. If the bone pieces can be repositioned by manipulation without any incision, the procedure is called a "closed reduction," a formal term that means the same as "setting a fracture."

Some fractures will stay put after they are set, and some will not. External casts or splints may give adequate protection to the ones that will. Sometimes a temporary period of "traction," pulling on the bone through a steel pin that passes through the bone, is necessary to overcome the tendency for muscles to pull the fracture out of place.

Closed reductions, casts, and traction are not the best treatment for certain fractures. If closed treatment is not likely to give a desirable result, the physician may advise "open reduction." Open reduction means that a surgical incision is made so the fracture can be reduced. Open reduction is most often combined with the insertion of some type of device to hold the bone pieces internally in adequate position, a procedure called "internal fixation." The combination of open reduction and internal fixation is sometimes abbreviated ORIF.

Fracture pieces grow together to restore the integrity of the bone, a process called "union." Fractures become united by forming new bone, called "callus." Once the callus takes on the characteristics of normal bone, the union is said to be "mature." A "fibrous union" occurs when bone pieces hang together by scar tissue instead of mature bone. Failure to form a solid bone bridge across the fracture site is also called a "nonunion." If union has not occurred in the expected time, but the physician predicts that union is on the way, it may be called a "delayed union."

It is more important to understand the principles of how and why bones break than to memorize the vocabulary of fractures. The vocabulary becomes important if your doctor uses some of those terms or if you read material that includes those words. If you understand the principles, you can usually figure out what the words mean, and you can always ask for an explanation or look the words up. If you have a visual image of what happens to bones when they break, the words will fall into place rather easily.

9

Treating Broken Bones

BROKEN BONES are a common problem in all societies. Characteristics of the population determine which bones break most often. Almost all of the people at risk for fractures caused by osteoporosis are over thirty-five years of age. A 1964 British study estimated the frequency of broken bones among people over thirty-five as being about one broken bone for each one hundred people each year.

If we consider every type of fracture in a population that includes all the people over thirty-five, we find no great differences in the fracture rates at different ages. That is because the number of broken bones from more violent injuries suffered by younger people balances the number of fractures from trivial injuries to fragile bones of older people. The number of fractures of fingers and toes, common to younger people in sports and industrial accidents, balances the number of fractures of the hips and spines of older people. However, when we examine the rates of fracture among certain groups within the population, such as groups selected by age and sex, we find some remarkable differences as to who breaks which bones at what ages.

When we separate women from men in the British study, we see some patterns of fracture occurrence that were not apparent in statistics for the whole population. People of both sexes sustain fractures at the yearly rate of about one hundred for each ten thousand people (an easier figure to use for comparisons than the one per one hundred cited above). Women at age thirty-five break bones at a rate of about thirty-five per ten thousand people per year, whereas at age eighty-five the rate for women is about four hundred fractures per ten thousand people per year. The rate of fractures for men actually decreases between ages fifty-five and seventy-five, then slowly rises.

Most broken bones in older people are caused by falls from the feet. Older people fall more often for several reasons, but the falls that break their bones would not have broken them when they were younger. The patterns of which specific bones break— and how they break—are unique in the older age groups. Older people do not have high incidences of certain fractures and unique patterns of fracture just because they fall a great deal. Falls may contribute to the problem, but they do not explain it: osteoporosis explains it. The bones of older people break because they are less dense than those of younger people. Older women break bones more than older men because women develop more severe osteoporosis.

The patterns of where bones break in older people are also explained by osteoporosis. The middles of long bones have small diameters and thick walls. The ends of long bones are much wider, but the outer shells are thinner near the ends. Because the outer walls are thinner, the ends depend upon inner trabecular beams to resist compression forces.

If you held a long bone, like a chicken leg, in your hands and were asked to break it, you would break it in the middle. If you had not already learned what you have about human bones, you might guess that they too would usually break in the middle. In fact, young, strong bones often do break in the middle when violently injured. Old, osteoporotic bones, however, are more likely to break at their ends. Fractures of the adult radius, for example, are one hundred times more likely to occur at the wrist than at the mid-forearm. The end of the radius is more susceptible to becoming dangerously weak from osteoporosis, and falls on the outstretched hand produce compression forces that cause trabecular bone to collapse.

Broken bones occur more often in people whose bones are less dense than normal: doctors knew that before they had machines to measure bone density. The machines have proven the correlation, up to a point. If density were the only factor, we would know that everybody whose bone density fell below a certain level would have fractures and that everyone whose bones were more dense than that threshold level would not have fractures. Such is not the case.

Occurrence of injury explains some of the difference. Even minor falls can produce major stresses on bones. Some people whose bones are not dense enough escape fractures simply because they escape injury. Another, and better, explanation is that measurements of density do not measure all the fracture-resisting strengths of a bone. Density correlates with a bone's mineral content. The cells and collagen of bone also contribute to strength. Elasticity provided by the nonmineral portion of bone keeps bones from being too brittle. The design of a bone, both of its internal structure and its external form, is an important determinant of strength. External support from muscle and other soft tissue also helps resist fracture.

Certain fractures become increasingly common with age because they reproduce themselves. Once you have sustained an osteoporotic fracture, the chance you will sustain another in the future becomes greater. The first fracture may be just a harbinger of the fact that your bones are weak enough to fracture from trivial injury. There is often more reason than that. The treatment, enforced inactivity, residual limitations, and psychological and social effects of a first fracture all can increase the likelihood of a second.

You cannot understand the effects of fractures and the purpose of fracture treatments unless you have some knowledge of the anatomy of the skeleton. Since certain bones and certain parts of those bones are particularly vulnerable to fracture from osteoporosis, you need to learn some facts about the shapes, structure, and names of those bones. Most of the pertinent anatomy is simple and easy to correlate with what you can see externally.

BONE ANATOMY

Bones form the solid framework of the body. They join one another at joints, where they are tethered by ligaments. The bony skeleton contributes a definite shape to the body, protects the more delicate organs, and provides origin and insertion sites for muscles.

Bones of the upper arm, forearm, thigh, and lower leg are called long bones for obvious reasons; the pelvis, shoulder blade, and skull are considered flat bones; and the hands and feet are composed of short bones. Some bones, such as the vertebrae and ribs, do not fit easily into any category. Bones that are within tendons, not connected by ligaments to other bones, are called sesamoid bones; the best-known sesamoid bone is the kneecap (patella).

For the purpose of understanding the problems caused by osteoporosis, we can conveniently ignore many bones. The short bones of the hands and feet seldom fracture due to osteoporosis. The flat bones of the skull and shoulder blade are uncommon sites of osteoporotic fracture. The vertebrae deserve special attention, but we can all but ignore the vertebrae of the neck and concentrate on those in the chest (dorsal or thoracic) spine and those in the lower back (lumbar spine and sacrum). The patella is the only pertinent sesamoid bone. Therefore, we must direct our attention to the dorsal and lumbar vertebrae, ribs, pelvis, patella, and the six long bones, all of which are vulnerable to osteoporotic fracture.

Ribs are long, flat bones that are held to the spine in back by ligaments. In the front they are composed of cartilage, which is more elastic and less mineralized than bone. There are twelve pairs of ribs: the upper seven pairs join the breastbone in front; the eighth, ninth, and tenth rib cartilages blend in with the cartilages of the ribs above them; and the eleventh and twelfth ribs are free in front. Together the ribs form a cage, the thorax, which encloses and protects the lungs and heart.

Thoracic vertebrae, also called "dorsal vertebrae," are the twelve vertebrae of the spine to which the ribs are attached. Thoracic vertebrae connect to ribs and to each other at two "facet" joints in back and at intervertebral discs in front. The thoracic spine forms a gentle curve with the convex side to the back, forming a roundness called the "dorsal kyphosis." The angle between the top and the bottom thoracic vertebrae is less than forty-five degrees in normal people. When the angle exceeds forty-five degrees, as it often does in people with osteoporosis, the kyphosis is excessive.

The front, or anterior, parts of vertebrae are roughly cube shaped. The blocklike front part of a vertebra is called the "vertebral body," or "centrum." Each vertebra is a complicated bone that forms a circle surrounding the spinal cord and nerves. The vertebral body is the deepest part, least accessible from the surface; it is the only part that people with osteoporosis are likely to injure.

Lumbar vertebrae form the spine from the chest to the pelvis. Lumbar vertebrae have shapes that are similar to thoracic vertebrae, but they have no sites of attachment for ribs. The lumbar spine is also curved, but in a direction opposite to that of the dorsal spine. The curvature of the lumbar spine is convex toward the front, producing a sway to the lower back, called the "lumbar lordosis."

The junction between the thoracic spine and the lumbar spine, the "thoracolumbar junction," is a site of special concern. Ribs tether the structures of the thorax, so the whole thoracic cage moves together. The lumbar vertebrae are more individual. Since all twelve thoracic vertebrae may act as one long unit, an unusual amount of stress occurs at the end of the thoracic spine

COMMON SITES
OF FRACTURES DUE TO OSTEOPOROSIS

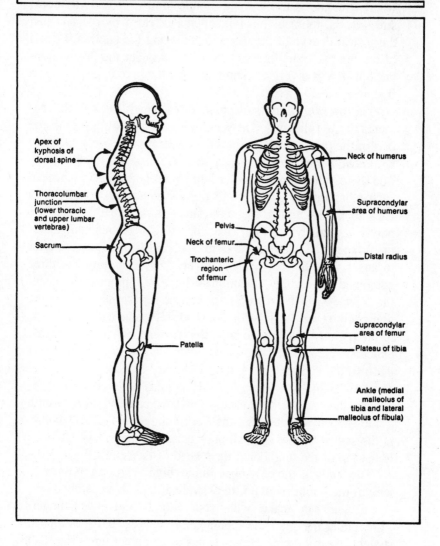

Apex of
kyphosis of
dorsal spine

Thoracolumbar
junction
(lower thoracic
and upper lumbar
vertebrae)

Sacrum

Patella

Pelvis

Neck of femur

Trochanteric
region
of femur

Neck of humerus

Supracondylar
area of humerus

Distal radius

Supracondylar
area of femur

Plateau of tibia

Ankle (medial
malleolus of
tibia and lateral
malleolus of fibula)

where it connects to the more mobile lumbar spine. Additional stress to the thoracolumbar junction is created by the fact that the forward curve of the thoracic spine and the backward curve of the lumbar spine intersect there. No wonder the thoracolumbar junction is a very common site of osteoporotic compression fractures.

The *sacrum* is the solid base upon which the mobile segments of the spine rest. The sacrum is both part of the spine and part of the pelvis, and provides the connection between the two.

Pelvic bones, three on each side, are separate in childhood. The three bones grow together into single bones that connect to each other in front by a tough fibrous hinge. They connect in back to the sacrum at the right and left sacroiliac joints. The pelvis is actually a region (like the thorax or abdomen) rather than a specific bone, but the term "pelvis" is often used to refer to any site in the pelvic bones. The proper name of the three conjoined bones, the "innominate bone" (appropriately meaning "bone with no name"), is almost never used. When the nonspecific term "pelvis" is not used, reference is usually made to the region of the pelvic bone that corresponds to the separate childhood part of the bone—the "ilium" is the large winged part upon which your belt rests; the "ischium" is what you sit upon; and the "pubis" is where your pelvis joins in front.

The three segments of each pelvic bone come together to form a cup-shaped socket called the "acetabulum." The acetabulum is the socket part of the ball-and-socket hip joint. The ball part is the top of the thighbone, the "head of the femur."

The *femur* is the only bone in the thigh. Through most of its length, the femur is round, thick-walled, and about as big as the circle you can make with your thumb and index finger. Throughout the shaft the femur gently curves, but it is almost straight. Near the hip, the femur makes an abrupt turn. The shaft bends and continues on up to the ball-like head as the "neck of the femur." There is a one-hundred-thirty-five-degree angle between the neck and the shaft of the femur.

Near the junction of neck and shaft are two bony knobs where powerful hip muscles attach. The largest knob, the "greater trochanter," is on the outside, where you can feel it with your fingertips when you place the base of your palm at your waist. The smaller knob, the "lesser trochanter," is deep on the inside. A line drawn between the two trochanters, called the "intertrochanteric line," cuts across the angle between the shaft and neck of the femur. The inter-trochanteric line and the neck of the femur are the sites where the upper femur breaks.

Near the knee, the shaft of the femur broadens and forms two knuckles of bone called condyles. The ends of the condyles contain smooth, slick cartilage that provides a low-friction joint surface for the knee. The area just above the condyles, where the shaft is wide and the walls are thin, is called the "supracondylar" region of the femur.

The kneecap, or *patella,* glides in a groove between the two condyles of your femur. The patella is encased by the tendon of the muscles of the front of the thigh. The tendon narrows below the knee, where it attaches to the upper portion of the lower leg. When you bend your knee, the patella is pulled through the groove between the femoral condyles.

The femoral condyles roll over the surface of the top of the *tibia,* the larger of the two bones between your knee and ankle. Like the other long bones, the tibia is smaller in diameter and thicker-walled in its mid-portion. The shaft of the tibia is wider near the knee. The top surfaces of the tibia are very flat, resembling high plateaus. Each side of the top of the tibia is called a "tibial plateau." The tibia is also wider at its lower end, though not so much so as at the knee. The lower end of the tibia is almost flat. Since the lower surface faces downward and provides the roof of the ankle joint, the flat, lower surface of the tibia is called the "plafond," which means ceiling. Along the inside of the ankle a knob of bone, the "medial malleolus," projects downward below the tibial plafond. The medial malleolus provides an inside wall for the ankle joint.

The *fibula* is the smaller, companion bone to the tibia. The fibula is only slightly wider at its upper and lower ends than it is in its shaft. The top of the fibula does not make contact with the femur and contributes to the knee only as a site where muscles and ligaments attach. The lower end of the fibula is more important. The outer wall of the ankle joint is formed by the downward-projecting "lateral malleolus" of the fibula. When you look at your ankle, the bone prominences you see are the medial and lateral malleoli.

The *humerus* is the long bone that connects the shoulder to the elbow. At the shoulder, the "head" of the humerus is bulb-shaped. The thin-walled bulb narrows, at the neck of the humerus, into a shaft of narrower diameter and thicker walls. The lower end of the humerus fans out into two condyles, and the area just above the elbow is the "supracondylar" area.

Cup your hand around the back of your opposite elbow; the bones at your fingertips and at the base of your palm are the condyles of the humerus. The bone that fills your palm, the bony knob of your elbow, is the "olecranon process" of the *ulna*. The ulna spans from elbow to wrist. It is largest at the elbow, tapering gradually to a small knob at the wrist. The far end of the ulna is clearly visible as the bony knob on the little-finger side of your wrist. At the very tip of that knob is a small projection of bone called the "ulnar styloid," which often pulls off when the wrist breaks.

The *radius* spans the forearm, parallel to the ulna. It is small at the elbow and big at the wrist, tapering in the direction opposite to that of the ulna. The elbow end of the radius is a small round knob, the head of the radius, which rolls on the surface of the outside condyle of the humerus. The head of the radius narrows very abruptly into a narrow neck. The middle portion of the radius is round, small in diameter, and thick-walled.

Near the wrist, the radius enlarges so that most of the wrist end of the forearm is composed of the radius. The radius provides almost all of the joint surface of the forearm side of the wrist. The tendons that connect the muscles of the forearm to the hand pass through grooves in the radius.

The far end of the radius is an extremely important patch of anatomy when one considers broken bones. Paradoxically, there is no unique term to designate this commonly broken segment of bone. The terms "distal," meaning away from the center of the body, and "proximal," meaning near the center of the body, are often used by surgeons and anatomists. The segment of the radius just above the wrist, which breaks so often in growing children and osteoporotic adults, is simply called the "distal radius."

HOW TO PREVENT FRACTURES

The discussion of bone anatomy just presented highlights the anatomical sites pertinent to osteoporosis. Many bones were not mentioned even though they are common sites of fracture, such as the small bones of the hands and feet, which are often broken, but usually from injuries violent enough to explain the fracture of small bones.

Fractures of the radius, humerus, pelvis, and femur, all of them large, strong bones, occur most frequently among people over sixty, even though people of that age avoid violent injuries better than younger people. The reason for the discrepancy is osteoporosis. Prevention of osteoporosis will go a long way toward prevention of fractures.

People who already have osteoporosis can avoid many fractures if they prevent some less violent, but still dangerous, injuries. Most such injuries occur at home; most involve falls from the feet to the floor. Many people fall because they cannot see. If you have impaired vision, always put on your glasses before you get up to walk. Keep rooms and hallways well lighted, and place night-lights in low wall sockets.

Loss of balance is a common cause of falling. Some people, especially those who are taking drugs to control blood pressure, become dizzy and light-headed when they first stand. Therefore, arise slowly and do not try to walk until any feeling of faintness or dizziness passes. Talk with your doctor about any dizziness or unsteadiness. If you tend to lose your balance, do not be afraid to hold on to some supportive device while walking. Walkers provide the most support and safety; four-pronged quad-canes also help with balance. Walking sticks are some help, but crutches may be more hazard than help.

When the cold weather keeps motorcyclists and overly competitive athletes indoors and safe from themselves, my orthopedic colleagues and I stay busy because of people with osteoporosis. Hip and wrist fracture incidence increases in cold weather. People fall on the ice, but that is not the only reason. Most people with osteoporosis are thin and not well insulated from the cold. Falling body temperatures produce stiff joints and inefficient muscles, and consequently people cannot readily protect themselves from falling. If you go out in the cold weather, dress warmly and do not stay out too long.

Dress for safety. High-heeled shoes are invitations to ankle and other fractures. Wear cleated- or waffle-sole shoes on snow and ice. Walking sticks prevent some falls. If joint stiffness, poor eyesight, or hand problems make shoelaces difficult to tie, get Velcro-closure or slip-on shoes instead of walking around with your laces undone. Wear clothing that will keep you warm without tripping you or making you clumsy. Long underwear and hats provide great warmth without tangling you in loose overgarments.

Make your home hazard-proof. You might find shag carpet attractive, but it is not safe if you have osteoporosis. Be sure there are no hazards underfoot near your bed or on stairways. Replace surfaces that are slick or where rough areas may trip you. Provide your home with assistive devices that enhance safety. Put safety treads in your bathtub and other slick areas. Install grasp bars on walls where you may need them for balance or to help you change postures. Keep stable step stools and benches where you may need them to help you reach or climb.

Dogs and other pets are great comforts and sources of joy, but they are common causes of falls. Train large dogs not to jump up on you, and take extra care that small dogs and cats do not trip you.

Other preventive and rehabilitative measures that are specific to recovery from certain fractures will be mentioned in the discussion of treatment of those fractures.

HOW TO TREAT FRACTURES

If you break a bone, you and your doctor must consider some alternatives. Many treatments sound painful and distasteful, but the alternative of no treatment may be more so. The option of very aggressive treatment, such as open surgical operation, may sound ominous, but sometimes the alternatives are worse.

You must weigh what you have to risk against what you have to gain. The difficult part of that, in the case of fracture treatment, is that the option of having things the way they used to be is no longer there. Immediately after a fracture, many people do not really believe what has happened to them. They weigh the risks and effects of some suggested treatment relative to their health the previous day, instead of to the way it is likely to be as a result of the fracture. Having the fracture just disappear, with no treatment, is not really an option, but the psychological tendency to deny big problems may lead us to consider it an option nonetheless.

Most people want their broken bones treated without open surgery and most osteoporotic fractures of the spine, wrist, and pelvis should be treated by simple, closed means. However, many fractures of the femur, tibia, fibula, and patella are better treated by open means. When you consider some of the goals of treatment and apply them to the pertinent anatomy, the reasons that is so will be more clear.

An immediate goal of treatment is to reduce pain. Most broken bones are very painful; the pain is worse if the bones move at the fracture site. The bone should be held still until the swelling and inflammatory reaction of the injury subside. But while the fracture should be held still, the nearby joints should not be held still for long. The chances of recovering motion in injured joints are improved if they move early. Return to normal or near-normal function as soon as possible. Economics and convenience are not the only reasons: normal weight-bearing and muscle activity stimulates healing and prevents osteoporosis from becoming worse.

Most of all, you want to live through your injury. It may seem unlikely that a simple fall from your feet to the floor or ground could produce a life-threatening fracture. It is unlikely that the fracture itself would cause loss of life, but recovery from the fracture may entail risks that threaten survival. Bed rest is a substantial risk, especially for elderly people. Blood clots, pneumonia, mental confusion, urine infection, and infections from bedsores are all complications of bed rest. Even in the absence of bed rest, prolonged disuse of one leg increases the threat of a blood clot.

In the mid-1800s, surgeons began performing open operations to fix fractures by using metal implants. By the turn of the century there was controversy about the advisability of such operations. In 1912, a scientific commission in Britain concluded that certain fractures were best treated by open operation and internal fixation. Since then, the controversy has become more complicated. Technological advances of the twentieth century have led to hundreds of ways to fix fractures, both internally and externally.

Actually, there is no last word on the subject. Recommendations change in response to new information and also in response to vogue. There is still considerable room for individual variation and application of personal ingenuity. Often you must rely upon your surgeon to use what works best for him or her. The generalities that follow will help you understand the specific injuries and make informed decisions about treatments.

FRACTURES OF THE HIP   The hip joint includes a pelvic side, which provides the socket, and a femur side, which provides the ball. When we speak of fractures of the hip, however, we mean only those fractures that occur through the upper femur. Anything on the socket side is called a fractured pelvis. Fractures of the upper end of the femur are treated by open reduction and internal fixation more than any other fractures. Few physicians recommend closed treatment for hip fractures, except in unusual circumstances.

The first operation for the internal fixation of a broken hip was done in 1850, but the method did not become popular until much later. In fact, the peculiar anatomy of the hip made it difficult for surgeons to understand hip fractures until X rays came into common use after 1900. In 1902, an American surgeon named Royal Whitman reported that he could get about 30 percent of hip fractures to heal when he placed the patient's legs in a cast in the best position as determined by X ray. In 1921, common wood screws were used to fix fractures of the femoral neck. The method seemed good but failed because electric currents developed in the tissue fluids between the screws. A few years later, nonelectrolytic metals were used to make threaded pins and flanged nails. In the 1930s, internal fixation of fractures of the femoral neck became common.

The practice of internal fixation of hip fractures persisted because hip fractures, treated any other way, are terrible problems. The powerful hip and thigh muscles pull across the fracture, cause painful motion, and force the bones into positions in which healing is unlikely or likely only in a shortened, deformed position. Prolonged bed rest, inactivity, and poor healing led to loss of life for many, and severe impairment of the quality of life for those who survived.

Even in the era since good surgical techniques have been available, statistics about hip fractures have been alarming. Many reports indicate that less than half the people who break their hips return to normal function, 15 percent die shortly after the injury, and 30 percent die within a year of the injury. Hip fracture is said to reduce life expectancy by 12 percent. Statistics such as these appropriately identify hip fractures as life-threatening. However, they distort the picture for someone who has suffered from a hip fracture. Many of the deaths that contributed to those statistics occurred to terminally ill people who suffered hip fractures coincidental to their terminal illness.

People who have otherwise reasonably good health should not be alarmed by such statistics if they fracture a hip. Orthopedic surgeons who care for many previously ambulatory patients with broken hips are much more optimistic about the survival and return to function of our patients than those gloomy statistics would indicate. A 1980 Swedish study that reported a mortality rate of 4 percent in the six weeks after hip fracture surgery is much more in line with my experience.

The statistics that nobody disputes are those that identify the magnitude of the problem of hip fractures. Studies from Finland, Israel, Sweden, the United States, and the United Kingdom all document a sharp rise in hip fractures in women over forty-five. Among women over eighty, some studies indicate that 40 percent have had at least one hip fracture. Hip fractures are two to three times more common in women because women have wider pelvic bones, which place more stress on the hip; because women live longer than men; and mostly because women develop severe osteoporosis more often than men.

Besides the cost in pain, quality of life, and life expectancy, there is an enormous economic cost. In the United States, hospital costs alone are over one billion dollars a year for hip fracture care. Without surgery to hasten the recovery, those costs would probably triple.

The rate of hip fracture in women doubles every five years.

In other words, twice as many sixty-five-year-old women as sixty-year-old women break their hips. The doubling time for men is every seven years. Another way to look at that important statistic is that if, by using the methods we already know to prevent osteoporosis, we delayed the progression of osteoporosis by just five to seven years, we could reduce the enormous suffering, loss of life, and economic burden by half. Even if all the things we did to prevent osteoporosis and to prevent injuries did not work well—well enough only to delay the occurrence of hip fractures five to seven years—there would be only half the number of hip fractures there are now.

Most hip fractures occur at home, because of falls from the feet. Some hip fractures are stress fractures: the final event is just the completion of a fracture that has occurred a little bit at a time, so the fracture may cause the fall rather than the fall cause the fracture. However, many hip fractures are definitely caused by a sudden fall. Home and personal safety mechanisms such as those discussed earlier in this chapter could prevent many hip fractures.

If you should fall and have pain in your hip, seek medical attention immediately. Some hip fractures do not displace initially. You may save yourself much grief if you seek attention before the bones separate. Hip fracture pain becomes worse when you attempt to move the hip and especially if you put weight on the leg. The pain is usually in the groin, sometimes down to the knee. If you think you may have broken your hip, do not try to walk. Call your doctor.

A broken hip is not a life-threatening emergency, so you need not rush to an emergency room before calling your doctor. The call is especially important if you are not sure which hospital your doctor will recommend. If you have a broken hip, an orthopedic surgeon may provide your primary care, but you will need your family doctor or internist to assist with medical aspects of your care, so you want to make sure you go to the right hospital.

The hip usually breaks in one of two areas. They are quite close together but are very different with respect to the troubles they cause and to the treatments they require. Fractures between the trochanters, called "trochanteric," "inter-trochanteric," or "I.T." fractures, occur below the hip joint. Fractures through the femoral neck occur inside the joint. Because of the peculiar anatomy of the hip joint, there are some very special concerns about femoral neck fractures that do not apply to trochanteric fractures.

The head of the femur is almost spherical. It looks a bit like the cue ball on a pool table. Most have a diameter of a little less than two inches. Most of the surface of the head is covered with smooth, glistening cartilage that reduces the friction as the head moves about deep in the socket of the acetabulum. Like a round ball of ice cream perched atop a cone, the head sits atop the femoral neck. The neck is almost as big around as the head, so the taper between the two is brief. The femoral neck angles up at about one hundred thirty-five degrees from the shaft of the femur, so the neck is not directly beneath the head in the sense of being directly under the head in line with the long axis of the body. Imagine the face of a clock with the center placed where the neck joins the shaft; a front view of the right hip would correspond to the position of the hands at one-thirty, with the head at the end of the hour hand.

Because the head is in an eccentric position, the neck must endure forces of gravity and muscle pull that act to push the head off the neck. If you hold an ice cream cone at an angle, the strength of the junction between the cone and the ice cream must resist the forces that tend to make the ice cream roll off the cone. The femoral head is not completely enclosed by the acetabulum, but is enclosed enough so that there is some intrinsic stability; that is, the fit is tight enough that the joint has some tendency to stay together just by a vacuum between the two surfaces. The close fit is not enough to keep the ball in the socket through all the stress and motions of a normal hip joint. Strong ligaments provide additional stability.

One ropelike ligament, the "ligamentum teres," runs from the center of the top of the head of the femur to the center of the acetabulum. More substantial support is provided by the "hip capsule," a strong cuff of ligaments that extends from the edges of the acetabulum to the neck of the femur, completely surrounding the joint. Inside the capsule the joint is bathed by a small amount of joint fluid.

Some of the surface of the neck of the femur serves for attachment of the hip capsule, and some is in contact with joint fluid. Unlike most surfaces of long bone, the neck of the femur is not covered by a periosteum with a rich blood supply. The blood supply of the head and neck of the femur, in fact, is not very good. A small artery along the upper edge of the neck brings blood into the bone. A little blood from the lower side of the neck circulates up toward the head, and a tiny area at the top of the head receives blood from vessels in the ligamentum teres. A healthy head and neck of the femur receive enough blood to get by, but they operate on a narrow margin.

When the femoral neck breaks, it usually breaks where the head attaches to the neck—the ice cream comes off the cone. Eighty percent of femoral neck fractures occur in people over sixty, and 80 percent occur in women. The incidence of femoral neck fractures steadily increases with age.

The bone of the femoral neck is a composite beam. It derives some of its strength from the inside trabeculae and much of its strength from the outer cortical shell. A slowly increasing incidence of fractures with age is more characteristic of the statistical pattern of bones that break because of gradual weakening of the cortical shell. Fractures that occur because of failure of trabecular bone are often compression fractures—the bone breaks because it is crushed together. Spine and wrist fractures are typical examples. Because of the stresses created by the eccentric position of the femoral head and the tremendous forces of muscle pull and weight-bearing that cross the hip, femoral neck fractures often are more tensile than compressive. The head is snapped off the end of the neck rather than crushed onto it. The average resistance of the femoral head to being sheared off the neck by such forces at the age of eighty is only about 30 percent of what it was at age thirty.

Just as the femoral neck has some anatomical peculiarities, the causes of fractures of the femoral neck may be less than ordinary. Reports from England suggest that osteomalacia may more often be a contributing factor with femoral neck fractures than with other major fractures. A study done in Israel did not confirm the higher incidence of osteomalacia but did suggest that femoral neck fractures are often slowly accumulating stress fractures rather than sudden single events.

If the event that finally results in a complete fracture line across the femoral neck is not too violent, the position of the head may only shift a bit on the neck. The head may then settle down on the neck in a slightly different position and heal. Returning to the ice cream cone analogy, it is as though the ball of ice cream started to fall off one side, but you stopped it and pushed it down a little into a more stable position on the cone. Such fractures are called "impacted fractures" of the femoral neck. If you must have a fracture of the femoral neck, an impacted fracture is what you want because the slight shift of position usually does not damage the already tenuous blood supply to the femoral head. Ninety percent of impacted fractures of the femoral neck heal without complication.

The greatest worry about impacted fractures of the femoral neck is that they might displace further. Healing is a slow process, even in such minimally displaced fractures. Tremendous muscle and gravity forces are trying to pull the fracture apart. Minor injuries are likely during the healing period. Therefore, most surgeons advise that impacted fractures of the femoral neck be "pinned." A "pin," in orthopedic parlance, is nothing like the straight or safety pins you may have around the house. When a bone surgeon speaks of a pin, he or she usually means a straight, semirigid wire, like a section of a coat hanger, with a sharp point on one end. However, the verb "to pin," as in "pin the hip," does not refer to a specific device. Many different screws, nails, and wires have been used to pin hips. If the device is much larger, say as big or bigger around as your little finger, the application is more often called nailing than pinning.

There was once doubt that fractures of the femoral neck ever did heal. Sir Astley Cooper, one of the British fathers of bone surgery, said in 1834 that in all his studies he had found only one example of a fractured femoral neck that had healed. In the nineteenth century, examples of healed fractures of the femoral neck were rare enough to be exhibited in pathology museums, and experts argued over whether or not the specimens really represented healed fractures or some other bone pathology.

Sixty-five years before X ray, Cooper said:

I can readily believe, if a fracture should happen without the reflected ligament [capsule] being torn, that as the nutrition would continue, the bone might unite, but the character of the accident would differ; the nature of the injury could scarcely be discerned, and the patient's bones would unite with little attention on the part of the surgeon.

Cooper was describing impacted femoral neck fractures long before their existence could be proven by X rays.

In 1934, Kellogg Speed, a leading American orthopedic surgeon from Chicago, gave the Fracture Oration to the American College of Surgeons. His talk was called "The Unsolved Fracture." He mentioned the various attempts that had been made to drive screws, nails, ivory pegs, and transplanted bone across femoral neck fractures. The results of such attempts had not been favorable enough to lead him to endorse operations for treatment of these fractures. The treatment of choice at that time was to turn the injured leg so that it "toed in" and to hold it, spread apart from the other leg, in a cast that enclosed both legs and the pelvis.

The next year F. L. Knowles, an orthopedic surgeon from Iowa, described a device, since called a "Knowles pin," that is still in common use. A Knowles pin is a smooth wire somewhat bigger than a coat hanger wire. The diameter of a Knowles pin is about the same as the click button on the top of most ballpoint pens. Screw threads that hold the femoral head are present at the pointed end of the pin. The outer end of the pin is capped by a small hexagonal hub. The Knowles pin is simply a long, thin lag screw. Many variations of the size of the wire, characteristics of the threads, and design of the hub have been manufactured, so many devices of similar design that are called by other names are available.

In pinning a fractured femoral neck, the surgeon makes an incision over the side of the hip, just below the greater trochanter. Beneath the skin, muscles and tendons are split to expose the lateral (side) surface of the femur. The surgeon drills the pins through the lateral cortex of the femur, then directs them along the one-hundred-thirty-five-degree angle up the neck of the femur, across the fracture, and into the head of the femur. X rays are used to confirm proper position of the bones and placement of the pins. The surgeon never actually sees the fracture in the neck of the femur. The hubs of the pins protrude a centimeter or so from the side of the femur, but the rest of the pins are entirely within the bone. Depending upon the size and design of the pin and the problems presented by the fracture, anywhere from one to twelve pins may be used.

Long, thin pins that contact only thick cortical bone at one site have limited holding power. Most surgeons think pins are adequate for holding an impacted fracture of the neck of the femur, because the position of the bones already provides a certain amount of stability. The pins relieve pain and provide considerable assurance that the fracture will not displace. If the femoral head is not simply impacted but is displaced—broken away from the neck of the femur—many surgeons prefer to use fixation that is more rigid than that provided by pins. When the hip fractures farther down, in the inter-trochanteric region, pins alone are inadequate.

The peculiar anatomy of the hip is responsible for two complications that are not uncommon after fractures of the femoral neck: the fractures may not heal, or even if they do heal, the head of the femur may slowly collapse due to "avascular necrosis"—loss of circulation. Only about 10 percent of people with impacted fractures suffer either of those complications, but the rate increases to 30 percent or more among people whose fractures are displaced.

In 1931, Marius N. Smith-Peterson, a Boston orthopedist, described his experience using a heavy, nail-like device to secure fractures of the femoral neck. The diameter of the Smith-Peterson nail is about that of the ring finger. Instead of a round nail, he made it triflanged, with three spines running along the nail. The flanges made it cut through bone more easily and, once situated, it resisted rotational movements across the fracture. The Smith-Peterson nail is inserted in much the same way as one inserts Knowles pins, except that the nail is so large that only one is used.

Large nails concentrate more strength than small pins and are not as likely to break. The disadvantage of the original nails was that they had to be driven in so forcefully that there was always worry about pushing the fractured pieces apart or holding them in a position that would not allow them to settle together. Recent technical advances have circumvented those problems: screw threads on the ends of large nails allow the surgeon to squeeze a fracture together rather than bang it apart, and sleeves to hold the nails allow them to slide if the fracture needs to settle during the healing process.

If displaced fractures of the femoral neck are to be repaired, they must be reduced. The surgeon must manipulate and position the leg so that the fractured pieces are back in an acceptable relationship to one another. Before the 1930s it was common practice to hold hip fractures in place with casts that enclosed the pelvis, all of the injured leg, and the uninjured thigh—called spica casts. Complications such as blood clots, pneumonia, urine infection, and bedsores occurred more frequently from spica-cast treatment than they do from surgery. Cast treatments often failed because muscle pull displaced the bones in spite of the immobilization. Once reduced, therefore, most femoral neck fractures are held in place by multiple pins or a heavy nail or screw in any of many available designs.

Unfortunately, fifty years after Kellogg Speed said it about femoral neck fractures we must repeat his words: "The fracture is still unsolved." We can reposition displaced femoral neck fractures, and we have marvelous equipment to help us accurately position beautifully designed devices of strong, well-tolerated metals, but not all the fractures heal and many of those that do heal go on to develop avascular necrosis. All our skills cannot bring life back to a piece of bone that has died because its circulation was damaged.

One response to the dilemma created by femoral heads that will not heal is to throw them away. Simply doing that was advocated for a while around the turn of the century. A much more satisfactory modification of that idea was provided once some of the problems with artificial replacement parts were solved. In the early 1920s one surgeon tried using a femoral head carved from ivory to replace the broken one he had removed from a patient. Experiments with femoral heads made from acrylics and various metals led, by the 1950s, to strong and well-tolerated implants made from metal alloys. An artificial femoral head, called a "prosthesis," is a metal sphere built upon a metal neck that is elongated into a stem. The surgeon drives the stem down into the shaft of the femur so that it is held like a long-stemmed rose in a narrow vase. The neck portion is flanged so that it rests on the remains of the patient's femoral neck. Many designs are

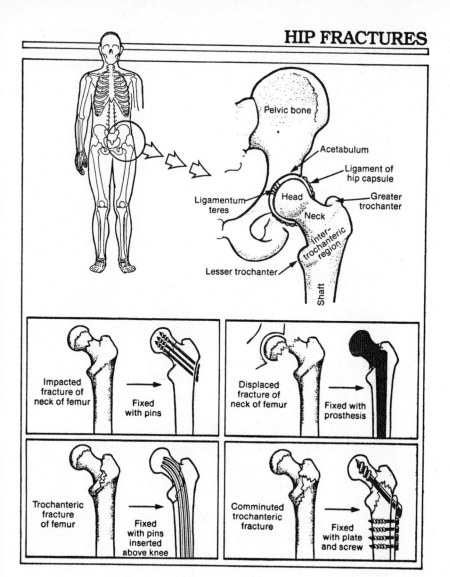

Pelvic bone

Acetabulum

Ligament of hip capsule

Greater trochanter

Ligamentum teres

Head

Neck

Inter-trochanteric region

Lesser trochanter

Shaft

Impacted fracture of neck of femur → Fixed with pins

Displaced fracture of neck of femur → Fixed with prosthesis

Trochanteric fracture of femur → Fixed with pins inserted above knee

Comminuted trochanteric fracture → Fixed with plate and screw available; the two in most common use, named for the surgeons who popularized them, are the Austin Moore prosthesis and the Thompson prosthesis.

The surgeon must perform a longer, more complex operation to remove a broken femoral head and replace it with an artificial one than to pin a fracture that he sees only on X ray. Not surprisingly, then, more complications occur as a result of operations to replace femoral heads than from operations to internally fix broken hips. The operation to insert a hip prosthesis is not exceptionally dangerous, however, and there are some real advantages to this approach to the care of displaced fractures of the femoral neck.

If a broken femoral neck is replaced with a prosthesis, it is not necessary to wait for the bone to heal. The protection, caution, and worry that accompany the care of an internally fixed fracture are diminished if you have a prosthesis. The reduced need to protect and care for the fracture is particularly advantageous to people who have other medical problems that make it difficult for them to care for themselves adequately. Replacement with a prosthesis obviates worries over fracture healing and avascular necrosis.

For many patients, unfortunately, a prosthetic hip is not satisfactory. The rigid metal implant does not feel quite like or act quite like a normal bone. The very best results from prosthetic replacement are not as good as the very best results from a healed fracture.

When a surgeon recommends a procedure for treatment of fractures of the femoral neck, he or she must consider some trade-offs. Ideally, the patient should understand and participate in the decision, but it is usually difficult for an injured person with no prior knowledge of hip anatomy to fully appreciate the long-term consequences of the different approaches. However, it is likely that as the problems of osteoporosis become more general knowledge, more people will understand and want to participate in decisions about their care.

A paradox exists in what is usually recommended to people with displaced femoral neck fractures. Those who are at greatest risk surgically, the oldest and sickest, are usually advised to have the largest and most dangerous operation—the prosthetic replacement. People who are too frail to fully participate in the aftercare needed to protect an internally fixed hip, and those who are unable to accept the risk of returning for more surgery because of nonunion or avascular necrosis, may be better off to accept the initially higher risk of prosthesis surgery. People whose activities are limited are usually happier with the result of prosthesis surgery than more vigorous people. Internal fixation of displaced fractures of the femoral neck is more appropriate for vigorous people who will demand much from their hips. They are willing to put up with the prolonged aftercare and the uncertainties of whether the fracture will heal properly, so they may have a chance at an excellent rather than just a good result.

If a femoral neck fracture fails to heal, pain will persist and the fixation device will eventually break or come loose. If avascular necrosis occurs, the hip will become painful and the range of motion will gradually diminish. If either of those complications occurs, one remedy is total hip replacement surgery. In total hip replacement surgery, a prosthesis similar to those used for acute fractures is used to replace the femoral head, and an artificial socket made from plastic or ceramic material replaces the socket. A total hip operation is a larger operation, with more complications, than simple prosthetic replacement, so it is not commonly used for acute fractures. However, when the joint is arthritic from an old fracture and failure of previous treatment, total hip surgery usually produces the best results.

Fractures below the femoral neck, in the trochanteric region, present a very different set of circumstances than femoral neck fractures. The trochanteric bone is covered by periosteum and has an excellent blood supply. Avascular necrosis of the femoral head almost never occurs from trochanteric fracture.

The trochanteric area is a wide part of the femur, supported by trabecular bone and relatively thin cortical walls. Because of a rich blood supply, trochanteric fractures usually heal: the problem is getting them to heal in the right position.

Powerful thigh and buttock muscles cross the hip. The muscles are held to length under some tension by the femur. When the femur breaks in the trochanteric area, the muscles pull the leg up and turn it out. In people who suffer trochanteric fractures and receive no treatment at all, the fracture usually heals (if they survive the pain and the enforced inactivity), but the affected leg ends up shorter than the other, and the foot points to the side, rather than the front.

Trochanteric fractures can be successfully treated by bed rest with traction holding the leg in proper position. Such treatment may require several weeks. The risks of blood clots, pneumonia, mental confusion, and bedsores make this treatment more dangerous than surgery. Such treatment may also be self-defeating, because while one hip heals, the other bones may become so osteoporotic from inactivity that another fracture occurs soon after.

When a surgeon places pins or nails through the outer cortex of the femur, up the neck and into the femoral head, the nail securely engages the head, but the hold on the outer cortex of the shaft is flimsy. When the fracture is in the femoral neck, the fact that the bite on the shaft is tenuous is of little consequence; but when the fracture is trochanteric, such fixation is totally inadequate.

Surgeons recognized that the Smith-Peterson nail is adequate only for femoral neck fractures, so they designed side plates. Side plates are rectangular metal bars with screw holes in them. Side plates attach to the nail and are fastened to the side of the femur with bone screws. Numerous blade-plate, nail-plate, and screw-plate devices have been made with many variations in design and metallurgy. The basic principles of all are that one part of the device securely holds the head and neck of the femur and the other part of the device fastens to the shaft of the femur.

Surgeons fix trochanteric fractures with angled hip devices, using procedures similar to that for insertion of pins up the femoral neck. The fracture is reduced and held by an assistant or a special table. The surgeon makes the incision along the side of the hip. The incision and muscle splitting are often a little longer than that used for femoral neck fractures, because of the need to secure the plate along the shaft of the femur (although many surgeons also use a short side plate when they fix femoral neck fractures).

A somewhat different approach to the fixation of trochanteric fractures has been gaining popularity in the 1980s. Instead of making an incision over the hip, the surgeon makes an incision just above the knee and cuts a small window in the bone at the far end of the femur. He then drives slightly flexible rods up the shaft of the femur, across the fracture, and into the femoral head. Since the fracture is never exposed, blood loss is somewhat less with this approach. A disadvantage is that the approach adds a sore knee to the problem of a sore hip. Many surgeons enthusiastically endorse this technique, but most still prefer the more direct approach at the hip.

Some trochanteric fractures are very comminuted—that is, very shattered. The combination of a comminuted fracture with osteoporotic bone means that sometimes, even with good surgical technique, the result may be less than perfect. "Subtrochanteric" fractures, fractures that extend below the trochanters, are especially unstable and cause concern about proper healing. The few trochanteric fractures that fail to heal or require more than one operation are usually severely comminuted, subtrochanteric, severely osteoporotic, or some combination of those problems.

Regardless of the particular operation, the results from surgical treatment of most trochanteric fractures are very good. Most patients can be out of bed the next day and walking with a walker within a week, and can fully expect a strong, painless hip as the ultimate result.

Surgical wounds around the hip usually heal within two weeks. Most patients are advised to walk with a walker. Whether some weight-bearing is permitted on the fractured leg depends upon the nature of the fracture and the treatment. When a prosthesis has been inserted or the fracture is very stable, full weight-bearing may be permitted as soon as it is comfortable. When fractures are internally fixed, patients are usually asked to limit weight-bearing for several weeks or months. Use of the walker permits a nearly full range of normal activity in spite of weight-bearing restrictions.

Because of change of routine, unfamiliar surroundings, and pain-relieving drugs, many elderly people with hip fractures become confused while they are in the hospital. If that is their first experience with periods of confusion, it may be alarming. Most often, the confusion spontaneously disappears once they are up and about and especially after they have returned to more familiar surroundings.

Using a walker to limit weight-bearing puts some unusual demands upon the upper body. Many people experience chest pain in their ribs and shoulder muscles from the efforts they make with their walkers. Upper-extremity strengthening exercises should be part of a fitness program to ensure safety of the lower back and legs. Arm strength becomes especially important when weight-bearing habits must change.

If you break your hip, you may need the help of a physical therapist. Once the fracture is internally fixed, you need to learn what you can do and what you must do to rehabilitate yourself. Most people can do much more than they first think. Physical therapists can help you learn to use a walker, cane, or whatever is best to help you with walking. You will also learn exercises to maintain motion and strength in your injured leg.

Many hospitals provide hip fracture patients with consultation from social workers. Twenty years ago that was almost never done; now it is almost routine. The need arose because of the confusing array of government benefits available, under specified conditions, to certain patients. Such benefits can provide assistance to people who truly need it; they can also cause harm both to society and to individual patients.

Many people feel, perhaps with some justification, that they and their families have paid so much into government programs for so long that, when they are due some benefits, they should receive them. That is all right if the benefits are beneficial. Sometimes people go to convalescent centers or nursing homes when they would be better off at home. Sometimes people clutter up their homes with hospital equipment that does not help them get better, and some have their lives cluttered by home visits from health professionals who do not really help. Convalescent centers, nursing homes, home visits, and medical equipment rentals are wonderful services when provided for the right people at the right times. Judging who are the right people and when are the right times is not always an easy task. Social workers, nurses, occupational therapists, physical therapists, physicians, and government service administrators all contribute their opinions. These professionals have individual perspectives, and often they want to dispose of the paperwork as quickly as they can while trying to keep everybody happy.

Quick answers and the approach of taking all that the government offers do not always keep everyone happy for long. Besides bankrupting needed programs, overuse of such services may discourage people from getting well and back to their own lives as quickly as possible. Fracture patients and their families need to consider the short- and long-range benefits and risks of such services before they request them. Often professionals encourage these services, but that does not mean that patients must accept them. You should understand what services are available, what they will and will not do for you, and what the costs to you and society are, and then make a responsible decision. Your responsibility is to get well, so you should accept what will help with that and reject what may get in the way.

You may be more functional with certain assistive devices

such as a commode extension, a mobile stool, and dressing aids for shoes and stockings. While you do not want to surround yourself with aids that make you look and feel like a perpetual patient, you do want to provide yourself with what you need to function maximally. Physical therapists and occupational therapists can provide advice about such devices and train you to use them.

After fractures of the hip, people must be especially mindful of all the personal and household safety measures described earlier in this chapter. However, they should not adopt a fragile, walking-on-eggs attitude. Internal fixation and support with a walker should return hip fracture victims to near-normal lives soon after the injury. Sometimes the patient's fears or well-meaning but misinformed relatives interfere with that process. If you break your hip, demand of yourself and those that help you that you maintain as nearly normal a life as possible. If you have fears about some specific activity or conflicts with a relative over what you can or cannot do, bring the matter up with your surgeon or physical therapist.

BROKEN WRISTS   Between the hand and the forearm, there are eight small bones that fit together like pieces of a jigsaw puzzle, but a broken wrist usually means fracture of the end of the radius. The small bones of the wrist transmit the forces of a fall to the flat surface on the end of the radius like a hammer hitting an eggshell. The end of the radius may be as fragile as an eggshell if the underlying trabecular bone has become weakened because of osteoporosis.

When you slip and fall, your natural reflex is to pull your hand back, stretch your arm out, and land on your palm; that protects your face or your buttocks, depending on which way you fall. By breaking the force of your fall with your outstretched hand, you may absorb enough energy to protect your other body parts from serious injury. If you then experience pain and swelling in your wrist, you have probably broken your distal radius.

The ligaments about the wrist are short and strong: they are not easily sprained. The forces that cross the wrist usually compress the bones rather than tear the tissues apart. For those reasons, after an injury a sore wrist usually means a broken wrist. If the fracture is not displaced, it may not look broken. Freedom to wiggle your fingers is no assurance that your wrist is not broken.

If you fall and then develop pain in your wrist, you need an X ray. Wrap your hand and forearm gently over a folded newspaper or any convenient splint. An elastic bandage is easy and comfortable, but cloth strips will do. Ice and elevation prevent swelling and pain, so fill a plastic bag with ice, wrap it around your wrist, and keep your arm higher than your chest. Call your doctor for instructions. Whether you need to go to an emergency room or not depends upon the severity of the injury and local health care circumstances. Many wrist fractures can be treated less expensively and more conveniently in the doctor's office.

A force that drives across the palm into the wrist strikes the end of the radius back of the center of the end of the bone. The piece, or pieces, that break off the end of the radius displace toward the back of the forearm. Look at a dinner fork from the side, turned back side up, and think of the prongs as fingers and the shank as forearm. The backward bend where the base of the prongs joins the shank resembles the shape taken by the wrist after most fractures of the distal radius.

At twenty-nine, an age at which most modern surgeons are not yet finished with their training, Abraham Colles was president of the Royal College of Surgeons of Ireland. In 1814, he described where the wrist breaks, the direction taken by the broken pieces, the consequences of the injury, and the proper treatment. He based his knowledge upon the visual appearance and feel of the injuries he had seen and upon his knowledge of anatomy. It was almost a century before X rays could be used to confirm his observations. Fractures of the distal radius are com-

WRIST AND FOREARM FRACTURES

Labeled areas are common sites of osteoporotic fracture. The distal radius is by far the most common.

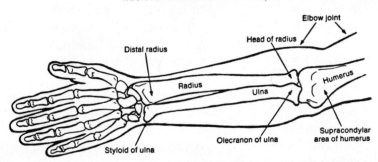

Elbow joint

Head of radius

Distal radius

Humerus

Radius

Ulna

Supracondylar area of humerus

Olecranon of ulna

Styloid of ulna

Colles' fracture

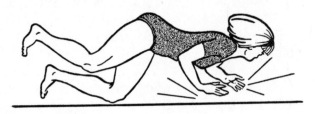

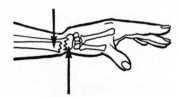

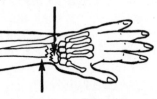

End of radius displaces upward

and toward thumb

monly called "Colles' fractures" (pronounced "collies," like Lassie and Laddie).

Colles described fractures of the distal radius that had displaced toward the back of the forearm, like the dinner fork. However, not all distal radius fractures take that direction. Two less-common variations carry the names Smith and Barton.

Some distal radius fractures do not displace at all. When there is no displacement, the aim of your first aid and the doctor's treatment is to keep it that way. A splint or cast worn for about six weeks will usually suffice.

When the fracture is displaced enough to produce substantial deformity, more treatment is usually necessary. Colles said that without treatment

the patient is doomed to endure for many months considerable lameness and stiffness of the limb, accompanied by severe pains on attempting to bend the hands and fingers. One consolation remains, that the limb at some remote period will again enjoy perfect freedom in all its motions, and be completely exempt from pain; the deformity, however, will remain undiminished throughout life.

Colles treated distal radius fractures by manipulating the fractured pieces back into their proper position and holding them there with splints made of tin and wood. He said, "The cases treated on this plan have all recovered without the smallest defect or deformity of the limb, in the ordinary time for the care of fractures." Modern surgeons, with all our advantages, cannot match those results.

Colles may have been given to some excesses in his descriptions, particularly of his treatment results, but the themes of his message have endured. Displaced fractures of the wrist cause pain. Patients find it difficult to maintain finger motion during the early course of treatment. The pain and the motion tend to improve with time, regardless of treatment. Changes in the shape and appearance of the wrist are permanent. Treatment by manipulation and immobilization improves the results.

A displaced fracture of the distal radius should be set as soon as practical after the injury. After several days pass, it becomes difficult to move the fractured fragments. In most cases, some form of anesthetic is necessary when the reduction is performed. Local (into the area of the fracture only), regional (causing numbing of the entire arm), or general anesthesia (the patient is asleep) may be used. The doctor may hang the arm in a traction device with the fingers suspended by Chinese fingertraps, like the ones you used to see at carnivals, or simply pull on the hand while forcing the broken pieces back into position.

Once the fracture is reduced, stability is usually provided by a plaster cast. Plaster was used to hold fractures in ancient India and Arabia, but Western man had lost the technique at the time Colles was using tin and wood. In 1852, a Dutchman named Antonius Mathysen convinced European surgeons to use plaster, and it has been used ever since. The one disadvantage of plaster is that it does not hold up in water, so in recent years plastic materials have been used in some cases. But plaster is still the standard.

The cast may be changed during the course of treatment. Initial swelling and fragility require that the first cast be larger and more padded than ones applied after swelling reduces and some healing occurs. The first cast often extends from the mid-hand to above the elbow. Sometimes the elbow is left free initially; often it is freed a week or two into the treatment. The fingers are left free throughout. A cast is usually worn for four to six weeks, then a removable splint for another few weeks.

A plaster cast cannot hold the fractured pieces in exact position. Muscle forces tend to pull the pieces back. If the bone is very osteoporotic, so that it is little more than a shell, there is nothing to resist the internal pull of the muscles and the radius will shorten. The shortening is limited by the position in which the cast holds the hand and by whatever bone substance remains to resist it.

In some cases, surgeons drill pins into the bones so the radius will not shorten. Using pins makes the treatment more complicated and introduces the possibility of some complications, such as infection, which are not likely during simple, closed treatment. The decision is made after weighing what could be lost by using pins against what may be gained in terms of preservation of the length of the radius and appearance of the wrist. In the majority of cases, no pins are used.

Shortening of the radius changes the appearance of the wrist. Pain diminishes and motion improves with time, but the change in appearance persists. The companion bone to the radius, the ulna, is usually either not broken or has only suffered a small chip at its styloid process. The length of the ulna, therefore, does not change. When the radius shortens it makes the ulna stick out more, so the knob on the little-finger side of the back of the wrist becomes more prominent.

The ulna is quite small at the wrist. When the radius breaks, the hand follows the broken radius and turns away from the ulna. A normal hand, when it is allowed to go limp at the wrist, will angle a little toward the little-finger side as it drops down. When a broken radius has healed with shortening, the hand will deviate the other way, toward the thumb. If the shortening is slight it may be noticeable only when the hand is bent down, but if shortening is greater, the hand can be seen to angle toward the thumb when the wrist is in a neutral position.

When the radius shortens at the fracture site, it often tilts backward. The dinner fork appearance can be permanent even after good treatment. The surgeon can reduce the fracture and cast the wrist into an advantageous position but cannot always control the movement of the broken pieces by simple methods. More drastic measures are not always wise. Sometimes it is best to accept the deformity and the consolation, as offered by Colles, that function will return and pain will abate.

From the time the fracture is reduced and cast, it is important to keep the fingers and shoulder moving. When the elbow is free, move it too. Stiffness and pain can be greatly diminished by early and persistent exercise. A physical therapist or occupational therapist can help you with your efforts to maintain motion. Some people, after wrist fractures or other relatively minor injuries to the hand, develop extreme stiffness, pain, and sensitivity to touch and motion, a condition called "sympathetic dystrophy." We do not understand all the causes of sympathetic dystrophy, but we know it is more likely to occur in people who are overly worried about and protective of their injury. A relaxed attitude, determination to maintain whatever function the doctor will allow, and early persistent efforts to keep the fingers and arm moving prevent sympathetic dystrophy.

The median nerve courses through a tight tunnel on the underside of the wrist. In the hand it supplies sensation to the thumb, index finger, long finger, and part of the ring finger. When the distal radius is broken, the median nerve is stretched, sometimes bruised, and often compressed by swelling. Tingling in the hand is a common but temporary result of trauma to the median nerve. Occasionally, the median nerve will continue to cause trouble after the wrist fracture is healed. Compression of the median nerve at the wrist causes a combination of symptoms called the "carpal tunnel syndrome." Tingling occurs on the thumb side of the hand. The tingling is often uncomfortable and sometimes downright painful. The pain tends to be worse at night, so people with this problem often awaken and move their hand about for several minutes to gain some comfort. The pain also tends to be worse with the wrist bent back, as when driving or holding a newspaper.

If you have tingling and pain in your hand after a wrist fracture, talk to your doctor about it. The diagnosis of carpal tunnel syndrome can be confirmed by a harmless electrical test of the conduction speed in the median nerve. Injections and splints sometimes help. If symptoms persist, a simple operation to release the ligament binding the nerve will usually relieve the problem.

Do not allow a wrist fracture to interfere with normal function any more than absolutely necessary. If you must temporarily limit the force you apply with the injured hand, you may find it helpful to outfit your home with such aids as doorknob extensions, turning handles for stove knobs, jar openers, and Velcro shoe and clothing fasteners. These aids are particularly helpful if you have injured both wrists or if you already had limited hand function because of arthritis. You must balance the benefits of forcing yourself to use the extremity as if it were normal against what help such devices provide. You may wish to consult an occupational therapist if you think such aids might help you.

You can prevent wrist fractures if you prevent falls. Follow the personal and home safety recommendations listed earlier in this chapter. Of course, you can also prevent wrist fractures if you prevent osteoporosis. One additional preventive measure worthy of consideration is the use of wrist splints.

If you have broken your wrist, your doctor has probably given you a Velcro-fastened, elastic wrist splint with a metal stave in it to wear when you first remove the cast. If not, you can purchase one at many drugstores. Some sporting goods stores keep them for skateboarders to wear to prevent wrist fractures from frequent falls. They are not expensive. A simple elastic wrap is no help; a splint must have metal in it and it must limit the motion of your wrist when you wear it. Buy a pair (they are made for right and left hands) and wear them if you are going out when it is slippery underfoot.

FRACTURES OF THE SPINE Fractures of the spine are very common in people with osteoporosis. About 20 percent of people with osteoporosis have only spinal fractures and no other broken bones; about 25 percent of people who have had spinal fractures have also had wrist fractures. Hip fractures occur about seven times more often among people who have had spinal fractures than among those with none.

When pressure is applied, the vertebral bodies crush down like a biscuit instead of breaking apart like a stick; they fail in compression. Therefore, fractures occur mostly because the trabeculae that support the cortical shells get too weak—the same reason that the distal radius and the trochanteric region of the femur break. In the spine, such fractures are commonly called "compression fractures."

In the vertebral bodies, 95 percent of normal bone is trabecular bone; the shells are not thick. Vertebral bodies are very vulnerable to loss of trabecular bone mass, a process that may occur rapidly at the time of menopause. Once there has been a reduction of trabecular bone mass by about 50 percent of what was there at age twenty, fractures are almost certain to occur. Fractures may occur from minor falls, from bending over to lift a roast from the oven, from trying to raise a sticky window, or from just ordinary changes of body position.

When the vertebral body breaks, it may form just a tiny crack not visible even on X ray—or it may suddenly collapse. Any degree of fracture may be quite painful. Sometimes when the collapse is not sudden, the pain does not begin abruptly. Many people have more pain a few hours or days after the injury than at first.

Pain from an acute vertebral body fracture may also be rather mild; some people have X-ray evidence of fractures that occurred without their knowledge. Many times, however, the pain is moderately intense. The acute pain usually lasts from one to four weeks, after which it gradually subsides. During the acute phase, movement may be so painful that there is little choice but to rest in bed for much of the time. Occasionally a week in the hospital is necessary if the pain is exceptionally bad.

Compression fractures heal; osteoporosis does not impair the healing process of bone. While healing of ordinary compression fractures is not often a concern, there are two big worries: recurrence and persisting deformity. Since all the bones of the spine are similarly affected by osteoporosis and vertebrae in the region of the fracture are under similar stresses, chances are great that additional vertebral bodies will fracture. Once a vertebral body is compressed, there is no practical way to restore its height, so it heals with a permanent change in shape.

If a sudden force is directed through the center of the vertebral body, the cortical shells at the top and bottom may implode. The intervertebral disc is forced down into the bone. Such injuries cause some loss of height of the front of the spine.

When cortical bone is not well supported by strong trabeculae, the weight-bearing forces along the front of the spine cause the vertebral body to collapse more in front than in back. More collapse in the front leaves the body wedge-shaped, with the short side of the wedge toward the front. Not only is the spine shortened, it is also thrust forward.

Forces concentrate and cause the greatest stresses at two places in the spine. One is at the apex of the forward curve of the thoracic spine, near the middle of the thoracic spine, where the back protrudes farthest backward. The center of gravity of the body's weight is farthest from the apex of the curve, so body weight creates the most stress on the vertebrae of that region. The other stress point is at the thoracolumbar junction, where the inflexible thoracic cage joins with the highly flexible lumbar spine. Osteoporotic compression fractures usually occur in the vertebrae near the apex of the thoracic spine or in those adjacent to the thoracolumbar junction. If a compression fracture from a trivial injury occurs at another site, it is highly advisable to look for some unusual cause.

Moderate-to-severe pain from an acute compression fracture usually subsides within four weeks. The fracture is usually well healed by eight weeks, but a less-severe, chronic pain may persist for six to twelve months even if no new fractures occur. The reasons for chronic pain after fracture are not all clear but can be at least partially explained by the change in shape of the spine, which places a whole new set of muscle and ligament stresses on the back. Compression fractures can cause people to lose as much as two inches of height in a period of weeks. Many peo-

COMPRESSION FRACTURE OF SPINE

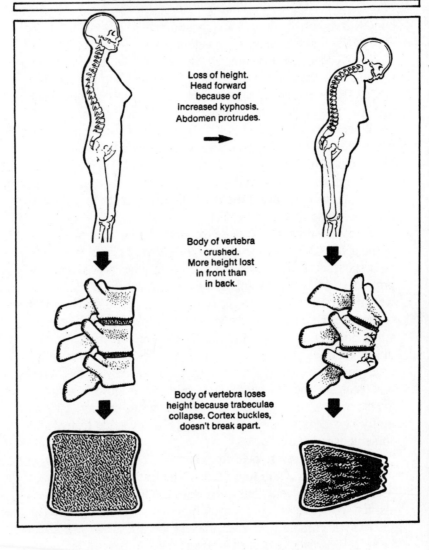

Loss of height.
Head forward
because of
increased kyphosis.
Abdomen protrudes.

Body of vertebra
crushed.
More height lost
in front than
in back.

Body of vertebra loses
height because trabeculae
collapse. Cortex buckles,
doesn't break apart.

ple sustain four or more such fractures and lose as much as eight inches from their height. The forward curve of the spine may make the abdomen protrude and the lower ribs abut the pelvis in front. The change in shape and loss of mobility of the chest may interfere with lung movement and impair deep breathing.

As terrible as the consequences of spinal fractures from osteoporosis may be, there is some consolation. People who experience pain and progressive deformity from repeated fractures usually do so over a period of four or five years; then the problem usually stabilizes. That may not sound like much consolation to you if you are not familiar with this problem, but it is to those who are experiencing it and fear that the repeated fractures and pain may continue for the rest of their lives.

Rest and mild pain-relieving medicines help you endure the acute fractures. Bed rest for more than seven to ten days is seldom necessary. After that you can get up for gradually longer periods of time, but it helps to lie down for about fifteen minutes every two or three hours. Once the pain from the acute fracture subsides, you will want to begin back extension and fitness exercises, as described in Chapter 11. Back supports and abdominal binders may also help relieve pain and support your posture. Many people expect too much from supports: they are disappointed when they find out that braces and corsets are uncomfortable and do not solve all the problems. If you don't expect too much, are patient with the discomfort and hassle, and don't depend upon it to the point of ignoring your need for exercise, you can benefit from use of a back support.

An elastic abdominal binder, with Velcro fastener in front, diminishes the pain of acute fractures and helps with the chronic, fatiguing, aching pain many people feel for months after a fracture. However, binders do not make you stand up straight or protect you from injury, and they do not take all the pain away. They crease and roll after you have worn them for a while, and they are uncomfortable in hot weather. But since binders are inexpensive, available in most drugstores, and easy to keep in your drawer, suitcase, or glove compartment, you have little to lose by wearing one occasionally. They are worth a try.

The next step up from the abdominal binder is a corset or support with staves. These devices are semirigid, so they give you more of a feeling of support, restrict your motion a little, encourage you to stand up a little straighter, and may give you slight protection from injury. Corsets are more expensive; some must be prescribed and fitted. They are more trouble to get on and off, hotter, and harder to carry around with you than binders. The top of the support in front may rub across your chest and irritate your breasts. Many people like the feeling of support they get when they first wear corsets, but they soon put them away because of the discomfort and the hassle.

Rigid braces made from metal bars or molded plastics are expensive, must be expertly fitted, cause a great deal of trouble, and feel very uncomfortable. They give substantial protection from injury and may help a great deal to hold you as upright as your spine will allow. They will not permanently straighten your spine. If your doctor thinks your spine is so unstable that you need a rigid support, you may derive some real benefit, but you will have to be patient with the inconvenience and discomfort.

Besides doing all you can to prevent osteoporosis, you can prevent spinal fractures by learning to avoid excessive stress along the front of your spine. Forward bending of the spine is called flexion. You can learn ways to handle your body that help you to avoid excessive stress in flexion. Good posture and proper use of your body help prevent spinal fractures and the deformity that follows spinal fracture.

Try to maintain the posture of standing tall. The shape of your spine limits how much you can stand tall, but most people can increase their height an inch or two just by adjusting their posture. When you stand tall, you also reduce the stresses on the front of your spine—the stresses that slowly compress the fronts of vertebral bodies and cause stooped-forward postures.

Imagine a wire coming down from the sky, attached to the

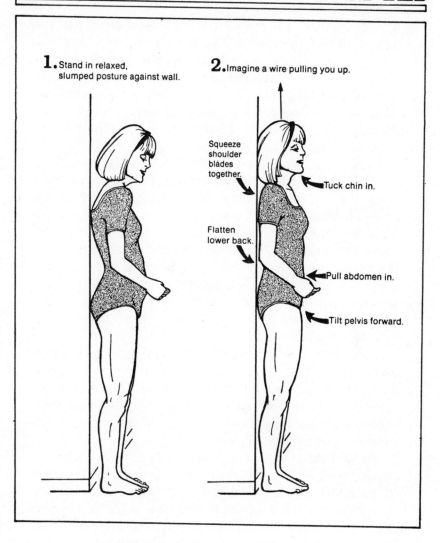

1. Stand in relaxed, slumped posture against wall.

2. Imagine a wire pulling you up.

Squeeze shoulder blades together.

Tuck chin in.

Flatten lower back.

Pull abdomen in.

Tilt pelvis forward.

top of your head, that pulls you upward. Now adjust your posture to go with the upward pull. Tilt your pelvis forward and suck your stomach in, and you will feel your lower back flatten and become longer. Imagine that you have a third eye in the front of your neck. To clear the way for that eye to see, you must pull your head and shoulders back and tuck in your chin, so your neck will become straighter and longer. Those are the postures of standing tall; make them a habit.

It is also important to learn to lift without straining your back. Before you lift anything, test the object to be sure you can manage it, that the handholds are sufficient, and that the way is clear for you to place it where you wish. Bend your knees. Keep your back straight. Pull the object in close to your body. Never lift a heavy object that is out in front, away from your body. Pull it in close and lift by straightening your knees. If you exercise to keep your arms and your leg muscles strong, you will be able to lift, push, and pull without putting excessive stress on your back. Exercises will also help keep your bones strong so they can resist what stress you do take.

Seek aids and be imaginative in avoiding excessive bending-over stresses. Pizza shovels may help you move foods about in the kitchen without bending and lifting. Keep your window casings clean and well lubricated. Use pry bars to loosen stuck windows. Use jar openers and other assistive devices so you can remain functional without sudden forceful efforts.

Spinal fractures may change your appearance. Do not let that change your life. You may need to have your clothes altered; if so, do it. Make your clothes and your surroundings fit so you are comfortable and not afraid to participate in life. If you need to cushion your chair to keep yourself comfortable at the table, do it. You may want to carry a cushion with you to restaurants. You may need to sit farther back in theaters so you can look toward the stage comfortably. Do whatever you need to do, but do not withdraw. Normal activities are important to your general health, to the care of your fractures, and to your efforts to prevent more trouble from osteoporosis.

OTHER OSTEOPOROTIC FRACTURES *Fractures at the Elbow:* Most falls on the arm break either the wrist or the shoulder. The elbow usually escapes. Elbow fractures related to osteoporosis may be across the supracondylar portion of the humerus; the olecranon process of the ulna may pull off; or the head of the radius may split. Muscle pull is so strong across the elbow and early motion is so necessary to preserve function that operations to reduce and internally fix elbow fractures are usually advisable. Minor fractures of the head of the radius may be successfully treated by early motion, but more severe fractures may require removal of the broken pieces.

Fractures Around the Shoulder: In British studies of fractures in people over thirty-five, it was found that the upper end of the humerus broke ten times as often as either the shaft or the lower humerus. Most of the broken upper arms were caused by falls. Among people over fifty-five, twice as many occurred in women. Osteoporosis of the trabecular bone of the bulbous upper humerus explains the frequency of fractures at that site in women.

When fractures of the humerus are very comminuted and displaced, the predicted result may be so bad that surgeons may advise internal fixation or even replacement with a prosthesis. Prostheses are generally not as successful for the shoulder as they are for the hip. Most fractures of the upper humerus are treated with a sling or light cast, followed by vigorous exercise to regain motion. Upper humerus fractures usually heal, but lost motion is a common consequence.

Rib Fractures: Ribs are long and narrow and vulnerable to injury by direct blows to the chest; it is surprising that they don't break more often than they do. Broken ribs may not show on X rays taken shortly after the injury. Pain with deep breathing and tenderness directly over the rib usually mean fracture even if the first X rays do not show one. Osteoporosis related to cortisone treatments and osteomalacia is more often associated with rib fractures than ordinary osteoporosis. Patience and support with an elastic binder are the only treatments necessary for most rib fractures, provided the lung is not injured by the broken rib.

Pelvis Fractures: I am usually delighted to be able to tell a patient with osteoporosis that the diagnosis is a fractured pelvis. The patient, family, and doctor are all afraid it is a broken hip, meaning a fracture through the upper femur. The pelvis is almost funnel-shaped, but the bones are much narrower in front than to the sides and back. Minor injuries most often crack the narrow pubic section in front. Symptoms from that area are pain in the groin with hip motion, pain with weight-bearing, and tenderness near the hip—easy to confuse with the symptoms of a broken hip. Fractures of the pelvis, when they occur from minor falls in patients with osteoporosis, usually cause little problem after the initial scare.

The back side of the pelvis hinges with the solid bone of the lower spine, the sacrum. A crack in the sacrum, which may occur from a fall on the buttocks, is difficult to see on an X ray. If you fall and experience persistent pain low in the back, it is possible that you have cracked your sacrum even if initial X rays do not show anything broken.

Healthy pelvic bones have tremendous strength. It takes a violent injury to break healthy pelvic bones, and such violence usually causes other injuries as well. Fractures of the pelvis in people with healthy bones are life-threatening. In contrast, cracks that occur in osteoporotic pelvic bones are usually minor injuries that heal themselves after a few weeks of limited weight-bearing. Therefore, everyone is pleased if, after a minor injury, the diagnosis is a fractured pelvis, because it means a happy outcome with no surgery.

Fractures Around the Knee: Just as the upper extremity breaks less often near the elbow, osteoporotic fractures of the lower extremity occur less often around the knee than at the ankle or hip.

The distal end of the femur may break through at the supracondylar level. Either plateau of the upper tibia may crush down. The patella may break from a direct blow.

Displaced supracondylar fractures of the femur and displaced fractures of the tibial plateaus are difficult to reduce and hold except by surgical means. If the displacement is not too great, it may be best to accept some deformity and loss of function at the knee and try to keep the situation from getting worse, usually with a splint or cast. If displacement is too great to accept, an open operation to reduce and hold the fracture may be necessary.

The patella (kneecap) is not directly connected to adjacent bones. It hovers above the end of the thighbone, supported by tendons. A direct blow to the front of the bent knee may smash the kneecap against the end of the femur, causing the patella to split or shatter. Very violent injuries, as when the knee slams against the dashboard of a car at high speed, may break any patella. The osteoporotic patella, however, may break from a simple fall on the knee.

If you fall or otherwise directly strike the front of your knee and you then experience pain and swelling, you should seek medical attention early. The skin is frequently broken from such injuries. If the patella is broken, too, early treatment may prevent complications.

Powerful thigh muscles may pull the upper fragments of a broken patella away from lower fragments that remain attached to tendon. Wide separations, if left untreated, severely weaken the muscles that straighten and stabilize the knee. Even slight displacements leave rough edges that grate along the groove in which the patella slides.

Undisplaced cracks in the patella are usually treated with a splint. Surgeons reduce and internally fix fractures of the patella if there is more than slight displacement. If the patella is shattered too badly, it may be necessary to remove some or all of it and reconstruct the tendon.

Ankle Fractures: Anklebones usually break from rotational forces. A turned ankle and a fall twist the ankle and the bones snap. Among young people, ankle fractures occur much more frequently in men, but among people over fifty they are twice as common in women. Among older people the injury may be a missed step in high heels, whereas a vigorous slide into third base is a common cause in younger people. The difference, of course, is osteoporosis.

Twisting injury to the ankle may cause an oblique fracture of the lateral malleolus of the fibula. The foot rolls out with the broken end of the fibula so it no longer fits properly with the end of the tibia. The medial malleolus of the tibia may break off at the same time. When both the lateral and medial malleoli are fractured, the injury is called a "bimalleolar fracture." If an additional piece pulls off the back side of the tibia, the injury is called a "trimalleolar fracture."

Displaced fractures of the ankle are sometimes called "Pott's fractures." Percival Pott, a British surgeon, described the injury in 1769. Pott said that such a fracture "gives infinite pain and trouble both to the patient and the surgeon, and very frequently ends in the lameness and disappointment of the former, and the disgrace and concern of the latter." Modern operations to replace and hold the broken fragments make outcomes from these injuries much happier for patient and surgeon alike.

Undisplaced ankle fractures can be treated with a cast. Displaced fractures can be operated on, reduced, fixed, and cast. Either way, early return to function, first with a walker or crutches and then in a weight-bearing cast, usually makes for a favorable outcome. Still best, however, is to avoid the whole thing by prevention of osteoporosis and injury.

IO

Psychology and the Prevention and Treatment of Osteoporosis

THE FUNCTIONS of our minds and bodies are not separable. Personality, experience, and emotions affect our bodies, just as disease, injury, and deformity affect our minds. Social forces, psychological attitudes, and situational conflicts cause osteoporosis, just as pain and deformity from fractures cause people to change their lives and their outlooks.

OSTEOPOROSIS AS A CAUSE OF PSYCHOLOGICAL PROBLEMS

Fractures cause much pain; they also disrupt lives with stays in the hospital, surgical treatments, and sometimes changes of residence. Some people who have endured one fracture become obsessed with the fear of another. Living in fear can interfere with the quality of life more than additional fractures. Living in fear can impede activities that help prevent fractures.

Even when expertly treated, fractures can produce permanent deformity. That is particularly true of osteoporotic fractures, because the trabecular bone is crushed and loses its form. Well-healed fractures of the spine leave people shorter and bent over. Fractures of the wrist change hand posture. Hip fractures often result in leg shortening and a limp.

Changes in appearance from osteoporotic fractures usually come at times of other difficult psychological adjustments. Many people focus the unrest they feel about themselves and their lives upon the visible changes in their bodies. When you think of the attention people give to such universal manifestations of aging as wrinkles and gray hair, you can easily understand how someone may become obsessed by a sudden change in height, gait, or hand appearance. Changes in height and spine posture change the fit of clothing. Hemlines may be too long. Forward stoop of the spine causes the abdomen to protrude and the shoulders to angle forward, making some styles less attractive. Furniture may no longer be suitable because the chair is too low or the table too high. Some people feel overwhelmed by those changes and they withdraw, instead of aggressively seeking ways to adapt.

Our hands are the parts of the anatomy that are easiest to scrutinize. Some people become preoccupied with the appearance of their hands. Shift of the hand toward the thumb side of the wrist, after a fracture of the distal radius, is more apparent to the owner of the hand than to the rest of the world. When we look directly down at the hands, the angle between hand and wrist is visible to us in a way in which it is seldom visible to anyone else. Some wrist fracture victims develop an obsessive habit of looking at their injured hand—a phenomenon orthopedic surgeons sometimes call "the oculo-manual syndrome." The oculo-manual syndrome not only delays recovery from wrist injuries and leads to complications such as sympathetic dystrophy; sometimes it causes people to withdraw from beneficial activities.

Changes of gait, limping, or the need to carry a cane or a walker cause many people more psychological than physical problems. Our culture is slowly changing to accommodate people with physical handicaps. Many people who break a hip were raised in a culture that was not so accepting of handicapped persons. When they become handicapped, they find it difficult to accept themselves. They may choose to withdraw at the very time they have greatest need to be active and to reach out.

TYPES OF PSYCHOLOGICAL PROBLEMS *Depression:* When unfortunate things happen, be they fractures, losses of fortunes, or losses of loved ones, periods of sadness are normal. Prolonged melancholy, feelings of helplessness, and loss of hope for the future go beyond appropriate sadness and into the realm of abnormal depression.

Brief periods of depression are common after many life events: postpartum depression after childbirth is a well-known example. Many people become depressed after injuries or surgery, but the understandable sadness and frustration that accompany illness do not explain the depression that often occurs after the critical aspects of the illness are over. Many people rise to overcome a life-and-death crisis and then crash into a depression when they are safely beyond the threat. Such reactions, when brief, should not cause alarm, but they should be recognized and treated if they interfere with a return to active life.

National Institute of Mental Health studies estimate that more than nine million Americans suffer from depression severe enough to require treatment. Clinicians who account for the people whose symptoms of depression are disguised as complaints of physical illness or self-defeating behavior problems believe the number of people with serious depression is much higher.

Depressed people feel that there is no hope that the future will be brighter. They feel helpless and unable to do anything to improve their lot. The facial expressions of depressed people are not animated. Speech and body movements are slow and show lack of vigor. Energy level is low. Such people may lose interest in food. Sleep disorders are common, particularly waking too early in the morning.

Depressed people may feel that their bodies are not right. They often have problems with digestion, vision, dizziness, heart palpitations, loss of sexual drive, and headache. While any such

symptoms can be signs of physical illness, they are often disturbances of function without any abnormality in the anatomy of
the malfunctioning organ. Sometimes an organ malfunctions in
response to psychological stress. Sometimes an overly sensitive
mental alarm system makes people interpret normal body signals as signs of disease.

Victims of depression may have crying spells, or feelings of
panic and worthlessness. They may lose self-confidence or be
overwhelmed by guilt and self-hate. Occasional thoughts of suicide occur even in relatively mild depression. Preoccupation with
suicide, plans about suicide, or any preparation or attempts to
physically harm oneself are signs of severe depression.

People who are depressed do not eat properly, and they often
do not exercise. Osteoporosis, therefore, is often a consequence
of depression. Since people who are depressed do not exercise
and people who do not exercise are prone to depression, it can
develop into a vicious, negative cycle. If it can be turned around,
a positive cycle results: exercise relieves depression, and as the
depression lifts, exercise becomes easier. If you can turn things
around for yourself, that is best. If you cannot, consult your
doctor. Depression can be successfully treated.

Grief: Death of a loved one may cause depression. Many of
the features of grief and depression are the same. In the case of
grief, the loss is often so great that family, friends, clergymen,
and physicians may not quite know what are normal and inevitable reactions to the loss and what reactions are excessive and
self-destructive. Grieving people may not know what to expect
from themselves and may fear for their future. They may have
no confidence that the feelings that overwhelm them will pass
and that the future holds hope.

Grief is a common human experience. It is especially common among people with osteoporosis, because osteoporosis is
most severe among women who are old enough to have outlived
their husbands. Although any one individual's experience of grief

is intensely personal, there are features of grief reactions that seem common to most people.

Grief reactions typically occur in three stages. The first stage of grief begins with the loss and usually lasts about two weeks. During this period, the grieving person feels dazed, overwhelmed, and unable to comprehend what has happened. Circumstances seem unreal, and there is a feeling of disbelief. The first stage fades into a second stage, during which there is growing awareness of the reality of the loss. Intense sadness and melancholy characterize the second stage. Many people feel an anger that they have trouble directing. They may feel angry at other family members, at the physician of the deceased, or at the deceased. They manifest a persecuted, "why me?" feeling. During the second stage, which may last six months, the grieving one is obsessed with thoughts of the deceased. Vivid dreams and hallucinations of the appearance or voice of the deceased may occur. These may be quite frightening, but they occur so often during this second stage that people who experience them should be reassured that such phenomena are part of a normal grief reaction and will pass. They are not signs of mental illness or hopelessness. The third stage of grief is one of reorganization. Morbid obsession with the lost one fades into a healthy ability to recall memories of the deceased and to derive pleasure from those thoughts. Confidence in oneself and hope for one's future slowly return. New activities and new relationships are sought. This rebuilding and reorganization stage usually occurs over a period of about a year.

Grieving people are most vulnerable during the second stage of grief. The transition to the third stage occurs naturally, and people should have confidence that the morbid preoccupations of the second stage will fade.

There are some dangers that people must avoid during periods of grief. Alcohol and other depressant drugs must be avoided. People should not be overwhelmed by fear because of the symptoms of their own natural grief reaction. Family and friends should be supportive and should not overreact. Persistent efforts to work through the problems of the second stage and into the stage of reorganization must be tempered with patience and confidence that time heals.

If a person knows that grief will pass, that life will go on, and that the future has possibilities, it is easier to maintain habits that will make that future brighter. In the depths of grief, personal maintenance may be difficult, so family and friends need to be firmly supportive. Proper diet, maintenance of calcium, vitamins, and other appropriate medicines, and regular exercise help one overcome grief reactions and maintain the possibilities for rebuilding.

Anxiety: While depression is the common manifestation of psychological unrest among the age group who suffer osteoporotic fractures, anxiety may have been the psychological culprit during the years their bones were being weakened by osteoporosis. The ubiquitous stresses of daily life in the fast lanes of child-raising, career-building, and seeking a place in the world produce tensions that contribute to the development of osteoporosis.

Many people feel they are too nervous, too strung out, too overwhelmed with responsibilities to make time for personal fitness. They deny the possibilities that regular exercise would not only protect their futures, but also would actually provide them with more time to perform their duties and leave them feeling less enervated.

Many people feel so stressed that they cannot even provide healthful diets and calcium/vitamin supplements for themselves, much less make time for exercise. The actual trouble and time commitment to provide the basics for one's health is negligible. It is the feeling of being too stressed to think about it that blocks most people. The price their bones (and their coronary arteries) are slowly paying for such behavior is exorbitant. If the advice of family, friends, or self-help books is not enough to control such stress, professional guidance should be sought.

Personality Disorders: When people experience the symptoms of depression and anxiety, they are literally suffering from psychological unrest. Many people, because of their genetic makeup, life's experiences, and current situations behave in ways that are self-destructive without actually suffering from symptoms. The results of their behavior may cause them to suffer in the future, but they are not unhappy at the moment.

The most important and most common personality disorder is the attitude that personal health is someone else's problem. We are all born helpless into the world and have strong needs for someone else to take care of us. With maturity, that attitude changes so that we may function independently as adults. Many people never mature with respect to taking charge of preserving their own health.

As children we trusted what we ate to our mothers. We now know that all the things mother thought about good nutrition were not true. We certainly know we cannot trust what television and magazine commercials tell us to eat. Reading reliable information about good nutrition is a little trouble; following good nutritional practices may be even more trouble. But what are the alternatives? Who is ultimately responsible and who bears the consequences?

The same lines of reasoning and questioning apply to exercise, smoking, and other health practices. Recognition of the problems and pursuit of the solutions are the proper responsibility of every mature person. Your personal health is not the responsibility of your parents, your spouse, your doctor, or your government: it is yours.

The invincible attitude is more characteristic of, but certainly not exclusive to, men. Some people think they can bully their way through life; smoking, eating high-fat foods, drinking excessively, laughing at exercise, and espousing a fatalistic attitude toward health and death are characteristic behaviors of those people. They often do not slow down to see the folly in their ways until some catastrophic health problem seizes their attention. By then, osteoporosis is often one of their problems.

An aggressive, macho style may be an overused generalization of masculine behavior. Its counterpart, the stereotypic menopausal female, is characterized as a nagging, unhappy nonparticipant in life. While such generalizations are patently unfair, they may be self-fulfilling. Many women grew up in a world whose media portrayed the middle-aged female as one who passively criticized and nagged from the background while doing little to actively improve her own physical and mental condition. Women who grew up to fill such a precast mold must count bone strength among their losses.

Phobias and idiosyncrasies can also obstruct healthful practices. Some people may be so afraid to reveal their bodies that they will not dress for exercise. Some people feel that exercise and sweating in public is undignified. Such Victorian attitudes are rapidly fading from our culture. Most people who force themselves to relax their inhibitions and try public exercise find easy acceptance.

AGE-RELATED PSYCHOLOGICAL FACTORS *Youth:* Young people believe they are immortal. They do not think realistically about their own vulnerability and their responsibilities to their future. Many of them are aggressively antagonistic toward any effort by the adult world to impose such values on them. Young people may react negatively to suggestions about such things as wearing seat belts in cars or crash helmets on motorcycles, or about not smoking. If health-preserving suggestions such as these are not accepted, how much more unlikely it is that children will pursue good nutrition and proper exercise, which are less dramatic in their effects.

Children may not always heed the warnings of the adult world, but they should at least be given the benefits of honest appraisals. Children do grow up, and when they do they draw upon what they learned as children to meet adult challenges. During childhood, they may not have practiced what they learned, but if the examples were there from what they observed of adult behavior, what they were told by their parents, and what they learned in their classrooms, they will draw upon those examples when they mature. Although it may not seem so along the way, adults are not wasting their breath when they preach good nutrition and exercise to children.

Menopause: The movement for women's rights is slowly eroding the Victorian precedent for the behavior of women during menopause. Freud characterized menopausal women as quarrelsome, obstinate, and petty. Melancholia or hysterical, irrational behavior was the stereotype presented to the medical profession and the lay public as well. As late as 1970, Hubert Humphrey's personal physician attacked the suggestion of a woman president on the grounds that women would not be able to make critical foreign policy decisions during menopause.

People grow to fulfill the roles that society sets for them. Millions of women were done the disservice of being taught that they would be quarrelsome and irrational when they experienced the menopause. Such prophecy accounts for part, but not all, of the psychological manifestations of menopause. Hormonal changes during menopause create uncomfortable and sometimes frightening physical disturbances for some women. However, education and intelligent medical management relegate such problems to the realm of controllable variations in normal human function.

The physical changes of menopause coincide with times of important life changes. Children leave home, marry, and bring home grandchildren. Husbands go through their own time of menopause, experience job changes and sometimes job failures. Many marriages fail, and women are forced to make adjustments in their careers or reenter a marketplace that is strange to them. Parents die. Friends move away. Much of the personality change once ascribed to menopause can easily be explained by reactions to such events.

Although many attitudes are changing, one Victorian atti-

tude has been reinforced by recent cultural change. The belief
that women should be retiring nonparticipants has been reinforced by the youth culture's idea that anyone over age thirty is
useless. The Western media's portrayal of beauty as having an
age of about eighteen, of exercise as the pursuit of sub-thirty
superstars, and of business success as belonging to computer whiz
kids reveals a society dominated by its young. This absurd dis-
tortion of the picture of power may make women who regard
menopause as the end of youth feel they are being encouraged
to withdraw from society.

Menopause can be a time of positive emotional events. Freedom from childbearing and child-rearing opens up new time and
opportunity for women whose careers were formerly pursued in
the home. By the age of menopause most women feel more at
ease with themselves than they were at a younger age. The freedom and personal power that come with age should be used to
overcome the fears imposed by outdated and ill-founded social
attitudes.

Old Age: Doctors have long been frustrated by their lack of
understanding of and inability to cure certain diseases that occur
more frequently among older people. Chronic respiratory disease, heart disease, stroke, Alzheimer's disease, and many other
medical problems that are now well defined were once written
off as "old age." People were told that such diseases were the
inevitable consequences of aging and that manifestations of such
diseases, such as decreased mental abilities and intolerance of
exercise, were to be expected among the aged.

We still do not have cures for all those medical problems,
but we are beginning to understand them better. We understand
them well enough to know that people do not cease to think well
simply because they are old. We know that people who do not
have heart disease have strong hearts and can respond well to
exercise, regardless of their ages. Artur Rubinstein, Eubie Blake,
Leopold Stokowski, Arturo Toscanini, and numerous other art-

ists have proven that people can be creative into and beyond their ninetieth year. Records for track events are kept for competitive athletes aged eighty and above. Freedom from disease means freedom to participate fully in life, regardless of age.

The medical profession is only partly responsible for the idea that people's lives are finished simply because they are old. Governments suggest that people beyond a certain age are no longer fit for the job market. Younger family and business associates push aside older people, using age as an excuse, when the real reason is the competitive, stressful nature of society. The media none too subtly suggest that the action in life occurs in youth. Older people are portrayed as impotent, fragile, and inactive. Many older people are impotent, fragile, or inactive because of specific diseases, but many others are simply victims because they accepted a role that society has unfairly cast for them.

The prevalent attitude toward sex during old age is a good example of the way erroneous social ideas rob people of pleasure. In an era of grossly explicit portrayals of sexual activity by the young, most of society is still embarrassed to talk about the sexual practices of the elderly. The Kinsey reports of 1948 and 1953 scarcely mentioned old people. Public information on the subject since has been sparse, giving people the erroneous impression that not much is said because there is not or should not be much sex among older people.

A Duke University study begun in 1953 has shown that, in the absence of specific diseases that interfere with sexual performance and in the presence of a willing partner, sexual activity does not decline until after age seventy-five. Many people remain quite sexually active beyond seventy-five. There are many reasons that sexual performance may be impaired among older people, but old age is not one of them.

An older woman may experience pain during intercourse because of tightness and dryness of the vagina—problems that improve with the use of vaginal creams and more frequent sexual activity. As a man becomes older, his penis fills with blood more slowly so it takes longer for him to achieve an erection; this is a problem only because of the anxiety it creates among those who do not have the patience and understanding to deal with it. On the other hand, many drugs taken for high blood pressure, ulcers, anxiety, and other medical problems may interfere with sexual function; diabetes, atherosclerosis, and other diseases may disturb sexual function. People who cannot function sexually should seek consultation rather than accept the explanation that it is just old age.

Many people accept the idea that exercise is not safe, not dignified, or somehow improper because they are old. Octogenarian marathon runners prove that such ideas can be wrong in the extreme. More important than those few superlative performers are the records of thousands of older people who have found renewed vitality from exercise programs. Exercise is discussed in more detail in Chapter 11. Some people must avoid certain exercises because of specific medical problems, but not simply because they are old.

Unnecessarily lost vitality in old age is not always because the media, or society, or someone else has imposed the wrong information on the older individual. Personal psychological mechanisms induce many people to withdraw from life when they have no physical need to do so. Fear of death is a powerful and universal human emotion, one with which all of us must contend in some way. As Dylan Thomas said, some people choose to "rage against the dying of the light," while others choose to "go gently into that good night." Those who go gently may unconsciously prepare themselves for death by withdrawing from life before their time. Gentle people may not be able, or want, to "rage"; however, if they recognize their fears for what they are, they may avoid premature and unnecessary loss of joyful participation in life.

FEAR

We have considered psychological factors as effects and as causes of osteoporosis, as specific diagnoses such as depression and anxiety, as reactions such as grief, and as manifestations of stressful stages of life. When we analyze all of that for relationships to osteoporosis, the common denominator is fear.

We do not teach our children as we should because we are afraid of their negative reactions to our efforts. Young people are afraid to consider their mortality and to risk nonconformity by adhering to good health practices. We are afraid that exercise will be unpleasant, that we may have to expose our out-of-shape bodies, and that we may fail. We are afraid of what society expects of us while we mourn losses and afraid of the rejection that may come if we reach out in efforts to rebuild our lives. We accept a living death of nonparticipation because we are afraid to face our own deaths. We are afraid to expect a great deal from life if ingrained, albeit erroneous, social messages tell us we should not.

We are afraid to ask for help. Doctors can successfully treat depression. Many of the diseases and injuries that interfere with normal function are treatable. Good information about nutrition is available at the library or from a dietitian. Clothes can be altered and furniture adjusted to meet changing physical needs. Exercise classes and groups are available or can be made available for people with handicaps. Before we can benefit from any of those things, though, we must have the courage to ask for them.

Do not be intimidated by social and media messages that tell you you should not or cannot do things. When you recognize the folly and injustice behind those messages, it should make you angry. Use that anger to overcome the fear of seeking what is best for you.

II

Exercise and Osteoporosis

Speaking generally, all parts of the body, which have a function, if used in moderation and exercised in labors to which each is accustomed, become, thereby, healthy and well-developed, and age slowly; but if unused and left idle, they become liable to disease, defective in growth, and age quickly.

HIPPOCRATES said that more than two thousand years before anyone clearly understood how exercise keeps bone from aging quickly. Of course, few people in ancient times had osteoporosis, because life spans were so much shorter. And those who did live long enough to have been affected, did not worry about getting too little exercise. Today, most people live long enough to make substantial withdrawals from the bank of bone they formed during growth. Since sedentary life-styles diminish deposits, withdrawals also exceed deposits. Proper diet and attention to hormone deficits reduce withdrawals but will not stimulate deposit of new bone. Regular, vigorous exercise is the only known, natural means of increasing bone.

Most people become less active as they get older. Older people tend to take on smaller physical loads. They make less-prolonged, less-frequent, and less-diversified physical efforts. All those cutbacks cause decreased muscle mass and strength and decreased bone mass and strength. The ratio between muscle and bone stays remarkably constant through life. You can estimate what has happened to your bone strength by comparing your muscle strength to what it once was.

WHAT HAPPENS WHEN YOU DO NOT EXERCISE?

Sedentary people experience a slow decline in their work capacities. Work capacity measures several body functions. The average sedentary seventy-year-old has lost about 30 percent of the capacity he or she had at age thirty. That includes about a 30 percent reduction in the amount of blood pumped by the heart, a 45 percent reduction in the amount of air moved by the lungs, and a 30 percent reduction in muscle mass. Regular exercise throughout life substantially cuts those losses, and exercises begun late in life can recoup many of them.

Studies of Harvard graduates, San Francisco longshoremen, and British civil servants all show that people who do not exercise are more apt to suffer heart attacks. Those at risk are not just unathletic people to begin with; the lower incidence of heart attacks among Harvard graduates was among the people who exercised later in life, not among those who were athletes while they were in school.

Rapid loss of breathing capacity and muscle strength are obvious to anyone who has ever tried to exercise after getting out of condition for even a few months. The effects on bone are just as rapid, though not as easily measured. Measurements of total body calcium show that people at bed rest rapidly lose bone mineral.

Weightlessness also dramatically affects bones. Astronauts on the Gemini IV and V flights lost body calcium at 1–2 percent per month. An exercise program reduced losses on Gemini VII.

Bone mass and strength depend upon muscle pull. People paralyzed by spinal-cord injury lose one-third of the trabecular portion of their bones within six months of the injury. Bones in immobilized body parts become osteoporotic. Studies of laboratory animals have proven the effects of inactivity on animal bones, and orthopedic surgeons regularly observe decreased bone density in limbs that have been held in casts.

Researchers have used ultrasound to follow the course of bone density in racehorses and humans. Sound waves move through bone more slowly after injury and among inactive subjects. Exercise training increases the speed of sound waves, a reflection of increased bone density.

WHAT HAPPENS WHEN YOU DO EXERCISE?

Exercise has subtle medical effects, as can be seen in accelerating ultrasound waves across bone, but it also has very human, personal effects. Exercise makes you feel strong and capable; it improves your self-image. It can be used to treat and prevent depression. Exercise makes you feel that you have more energy. Group exercise leads to friendships and social support.

In general, people who exercise regularly sleep better and eat better. Bowel function is improved by regular exercise. People who stay fit have a slower pulse rate and lower blood pressure. People who exercise also take less medicine—fewer tranquilizers, blood pressure pills, laxatives, antacids, and sleeping pills. Since the side effects of medicine can lead to osteoporosis, obviating the need for medicine is another way in which exercise preserves bone strength.

Injuries occur when people are fatigued and when they have taken on more than they can handle. Falls result from loss of balance and failure of coordination. Increased work capacity, increased coordination, and greater strength to prevent injuries are other ways in which exercise reduces the suffering caused by osteoporosis.

Beyond influencing general well-being, exercise has some very specific positive effects on bones. Experiments on laboratory animals, studies of unique groups of people, and observations of unusual cases all provide examples of how exercised bone increases in mass and strength. For example, a report published in the *British Medical Journal* in October 1950 cited the case of a twenty-three-year-old man who lost all the digits of his right hand except for the little finger. Thereafter, he worked as a laborer. When examined thirty-two years later, the little finger on the right hand was the size of the long finger of his left hand and much larger than the little finger of his left hand. The bones and soft tissues of his little finger had grown in response to exercise, even though the extra exercise had not begun until adult life.

A similar phenomenon was observed in a 1981 British laboratory experiment. Sheep were studied after surgeons removed their ulnas. Where the ulna was removed, its companion bone, the radius, slowly enlarged until the bone mass of the radius eventually came to be about as large as the combined mass of the ulna and radius had been before surgery. The increase in size of the radius was directly related to the amount of exercise the sheep were given, up to a point. More exercise enlarged the radius faster, over a very wide range of activity, although there was a limit beyond which more exercise did not help.

The shoulders of baseball pitchers, the forearms of tennis players, and the legs of ballet dancers all have large and strong bones. Tennis players have been studied carefully because some people play tennis for fifty years or more and because the nondominant arm provides a good comparison. The bones of the dominant arm of tennis players are thicker and denser than those of their nondominant arms by about 15 percent, whereas there is only a 3 percent difference between right and left arms of nonathletes.

A 1974 Scandinavian study showed that cross-country runners have unusually dense leg bones. Marathon runners do not lose muscle and gain fat as they age, and their bones are denser than nonathletes of the same age. The same phenomenon has been observed in laboratory rats given treadmill exercises.

Exercise strengthens bones in the spine, a finding especially pertinent to the subject of osteoporosis. A 1983 University of

West Virginia experiment showed that repeated loading of rabbits' hind legs strengthened not only their tibias and femurs, but the vertebrae of their lumbar and thoracic spines as well. Forcing dogs to carry lead weights strengthens the bodies of their vertebrae.

These observations strongly suggest that exercise can strengthen bone and should help osteoporosis. The hypothesis is put to the test when elderly women are measured before and after supervised exercise programs. Studies in 1980 at the University of Wisconsin showed that women in their eighties who exercised for thirty minutes at least three times per week gained bone density and total body calcium, while women of the same age who did not exercise lost density and calcium.

Older people can also increase their muscle mass by exercise. A 1977 Finnish study of people, average age sixty-nine, showed that muscle mass, muscle enzymes, and ability to burn oxygen all increased as a result of exercise. Muscle mass correlates with bone mass; strong muscle pull stimulates bone formation; and strong muscles prevent injuries.

While the ends of long bones stop growing in youth, the periosteal envelope that surrounds bone continues to make new bone throughout life. Thickness and strength of new periosteal bone depend upon the stresses placed on the bone. New bone from the periosteum and reorganization of the internal trabecular bone occur in response to stress, according to Wolff's Law, as described in Chapter 3. Exercise stresses bones; bones respond by strengthening themselves.

Bone health depends upon healthy circulation, and exercise stimulates circulation. Our bodies are filled with potential alternate pathways for blood flow. In a city, traffic flows mostly through the main streets unless the main streets are blocked or the traffic becomes so heavy that it becomes advantageous to open up side streets. Exercise increases the flow of blood so that secondary channels open. Increased blood flow stimulates growth of areas that were previously out of the mainstream.

Our bodies respond to exercise with hormone and other chemical changes. Though we do not understand much about the mechanisms, exercise probably improves bone health because chemical messengers signal bone cells to slow bone breakdown and speed bone formation.

PRECAUTIONS

Many older people are afraid to exercise because they fear a heart attack. People who exercise are less likely to have heart attacks, but that is not complete reassurance for those who are out of shape and afraid to begin exercising. It is naive to think that exercise is no risk: people have had heart attacks or suffered other injuries while exercising. Instead of denying the possibility of harm from exercise, one should make realistic assessments of the risks and the benefits.

For most people, the risk of not exercising is considerably greater than the risk of exercising. Most people who give fear of injury as the reason that they do not exercise do not want to think about the greater risks they take when they choose not to exercise.

There is certainly no harm in having your doctor examine you before you begin an exercise program (although one could make an even better case for having your doctor examine you before you decide *not* to begin an exercise program). And people who are out of shape, overweight, smoke, have high blood pressure, have a personal or family history of heart disease or diabetes, or are over forty should definitely consult their physicians before beginning an exercise program. In many cases, it is wise to have a stress test.

If you can take your pulse, you can monitor stress on your heart while you exercise. The easiest pulse to monitor during exercise is the carotid pulse, which you can feel by placing the fingertips of the opposite hand between your larynx (Adam's apple) and the long muscle that runs from the angle of your jaw to the top of your breastbone. To obtain your pulse rate, count pulses for ten seconds and multiply by six. Your pulse rate should never exceed 75 percent of 220 less your age—for example, if you are sixty, your pulse rate should not exceed $220 - 60 = 160 \times .75 = 120$. You may breathe harder than normal, but you should not be so out of breath that you cannot carry on a conversation.

Increased adrenaline and other chemical changes of exercise may cause trouble if you stop exercising abruptly. Sprinting to the finish line, then stopping to talk to reporters, may be something superstars do on television, but it is not safe. Always warm down slowly, doing easier and more relaxed exercises before you stop.

Everyone should know how to give cardiopulmonary resuscitation (CPR). Exercising with someone provides additional safety for you both if you both know CPR.

If high-performance athletes can suffer stress fractures, you may wonder how someone with osteoporosis can exercise without risk of fracture. Again, it is naive to assume there is no risk of fracture from exercise. But for most people, the risk of fracture from not exercising is greater than the risk of exercising. Injuries stress bones and cause them to fracture. Exercise stresses bones. Excessive and foolish exercises can cause fractures. Exercise should be a controlled stress—just enough to stimulate strengthening and not enough to cause fracture.

Select exercises that are safe for you. Exercise in a safe environment where accidents will not occur during the exercise period. Be patient; allow yourself to progress slowly. It takes a long time for muscles and bones to regain strength. Exercise programs should be lifetime commitments. Hurry-up programs cause only frustration and injury.

Women who train for high performance in endurance sports, such as distance running, may cease having menstrual periods.

As many as 80 percent of young women in such sports report menstrual irregularities during intense training. The menstrual cycle returns to normal within two months when they stop training. Some women who stop menstruating because of intense physical training have been found to have osteoporosis. Those are cases of extreme stress causing hormonal imbalance well beyond what nonathletes embarked on a fitness program would experience. These unusual incidents should not dissuade people from pursuing ordinary exercise programs.

Exercise helps most people reorder their lives in healthful ways. You may need to make a few minor adjustments in your routine, such as increasing your intake of fluids to make up for what you lose in sweat. Salt pills are dangerous and unnecessary; all you need is more water. Speeded-up bowel function may reduce absorption, so you should be extra careful to maintain slightly more than minimum levels of calcium, minerals, and vitamins.

When you assess your need for exercise, do not deceive yourself about your current exercise status. Many people believe they get enough exercise because their work wears them out, but few people work at jobs that really provide good physical exercise. Most people are worn out from emotional stress and lack of good physical exercise.

Likewise, some people are convinced their recreational activities keep them in shape. However, few sports really provide good fitness exercise. Many people count golf and bowling among their exercise activities. Golf, bowling, and similar sports are fine recreation, but they are not good exercise. In fact, for people with osteoporosis, the sudden stresses while bending over and the risks of a fall or an off-balance move make fracture risk higher in such sports than during controlled exercise. This does not mean that you should not participate in such sports, but it does mean that you need to supplement that participation with a good exercise program.

EXERCISES TO PREVENT FRACTURES

Before you consider specific exercise techniques, think about types and goals of exercise. There are hundreds of satisfactory exercises. You can choose the most pleasant and effective ones for you if you understand some principles.

Strength, flexibility, endurance, coordination, and posture are the five main goals of exercises for osteoporosis. Another goal, relaxation, may be important to the quality of your life, but it is not so pertinent to osteoporosis.

The components of an exercise are peak load, rate of application of the load, duration of each effort, frequency of repetitions, number of repetitions during any one session, diversity of movements, and frequency of sessions. Those components can be varied to accommodate specific goals and to fit your schedule.

You can build strength by paying attention to peak load and duration of effort, as is done in lifting weights that strain the limits of your strength. The goal of strength, in the sense of muscle power, usually does not require as many repetitions or as frequent sessions as do goals of flexibility and endurance. About ten repetitions at near-maximum effort, two or three times per week, will increase muscle power.

Efforts to increase flexibility require more time than strength-building exercises. Heavy loads at the limits of flexibility are seldom helpful and may be dangerous. Multiple (usually five to ten) and slowly applied efforts are best for flexibility. You should make efforts to gain motion at least daily. You might be more successful if you make them even more frequently.

Posture exercises are really special, low-intensity variations of flexibility exercises. You should repeat them throughout your day. Endurance exercises require multiple repetitions over long sessions, at least every other day. General fitness improves with continuous, high-frequency, low-intensity efforts of thirty minutes or longer. Once you have conditioned yourself, you can sustain rhythmic, repetitive movements, such as walking, running, bicycling, swimming, and rowing.

Coordination develops from rapid frequency and diversity of movements. Balance is an important component of coordination exercises.

Beginning exercisers and those who are trying to recapture lost fitness should exercise in groups whenever possible. Group exercises are safer. Also, groups are usually more effective because of mutual support and stimulation. Lack of access to a group is seldom reason enough to forgo exercising, but it is best to have someone join you when you can.

You can learn exercises that do not require special equipment. However, you can work more efficiently, particularly in exercising for strengthening, if you use exercise equipment. Free weights suffice for most purposes but can be dangerous for unathletic people. A recreation center or health spa with good weight equipment is ideal, if you have access to one and if you can obtain instruction in use of the equipment. If you have osteoporosis, you should ask your doctor before using any exercise equipment and pass your doctor's comments on to the instructor.

Precede any effort to push yourself near your limit with about fifteen minutes of warm-up. Easy flexibility exercises are good warm-ups. Warm-ups are especially important before strengthening exercises, because muscles and joints must be prepared to accept high peak loads or rapidly applied loads. Warm-down exercises are even more important than warm-up exercises. Tapering your session down with five or more minutes of easy, relaxing exercise is especially important after endurance training.

Arm Exercises: Move your hands up and down, side to side, and in rotation, as when turning a doorknob. Open and close your fingers rapidly and move your wrists through full ranges of

motion. Finger and wrist flexibility exercises are good low-
energy warm-up exercises. Follow them by working your elbows up and down and stretching your arms toward the ceiling.

Strong arm muscles prevent injuries. The stress of exercise
keeps forearm bones strong and prevents wrist fractures. You
can best strengthen your arm muscles with weights. Small
dumbbells suffice for most people and are reasonably safe.

Neck Exercises: Neck fractures are not common consequences of osteoporosis. However, neck pains occur in people
whose dorsal spines are bent forward from osteoporosis because
they must strain their necks in order to direct their gaze forward.

Move your neck in three planes. Bend it side to side, as when
you put your ear to your shoulder. Rotate it, as when you turn
your chin to your shoulder. Bend your lower neck forward and
back, as when you put your chin on your chest, and then move
your head back to look at the ceiling. Bend your upper neck forward when you tuck your chin in like a military cadet. Keep
your neck flexible by relaxed movements through full range in
all three planes. Tuck your chin in and extend your head a little
to practice the neck component of the "stand-tall" posture exercise.

Shoulder and Chest Exercises: Your arms join your chest
where your shoulder blades contact your rib cage. Your shoulder blade is a flat bone that glides on your chest wall. When
your shoulder blades glide forward, the weight of your arms falls
in front of your body and pulls down on your upper back.

Feel the movement of your shoulder blades by shrugging your
shoulders up to your ears, then letting them fall, and by trying
to pull your shoulders together in front of your chest, then moving them back. Move them all the way back so they pinch together in the middle. Pinching your shoulder blades together
in the middle of your back is another part of the stand-tall
posture.

Clasp your hands behind your head and draw your elbows
back, then take deep breaths; this will help maintain the flexi-

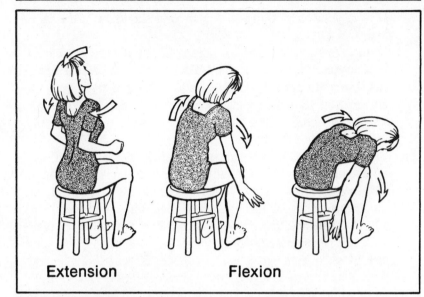

Extension   Flexion

Shoulder and chest flexibility

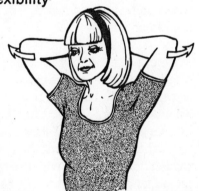

Clasp hands behind head.
Sit tall.
Pull elbows back.
Squeeze shoulder blades together.
Expand chest.
Breathe deeply.

bility of your chest wall and stretch your shoulders at the same time.

Back Exercises: Complex groups of small muscles, called extensor muscles, run in columns along either side of your back. Back strength comes from extensor muscles and from muscles that surround your chest and abdomen. Strong chest and abdominal muscles convert the spine from a narrow, serpentine column to a sturdy cylinder.

When you bend backward, as though to look at the ceiling, you extend your spine. The motion is called extension, and the muscles that propel it are called extensors. Bend forward, as though to touch your toes, and flex your spine. The motion is called flexion, and the muscles that power it are called flexors.

Strong flexor muscles are important because they support your spine by strengthening the whole cylinder of your abdomen and chest. Exercises to strengthen the abdominal flexors and to make the spine flex more freely must be approached very cautiously by people with osteoporosis. The forces of flexion stress the front of the vertebral bodies, where they may fracture if they are weak from osteoporosis.

People who do not have osteoporosis should certainly do flexion exercises. Stress in flexion stimulates the vertebral bodies to become stronger, thereby preventing fractures later. People who already have osteoporosis have a dilemma regarding flexion exercises. They cannot strengthen their vertebrae with flexion exercises because they risk fracture from the exercises. Those who have had recent spinal fractures should avoid flexion exercises. Some people with osteoporosis who are not in imminent danger of spinal fracture should cautiously begin some flexion exercises. A physician's advice may help with this difficult decision.

The best flexion exercise for strengthening is the bent-knee sit-up. If you lie on your back, feet flat on the floor and knees bent, and raise your head and shoulders up a few inches, you will feel your abdominal flexor muscles tighten. There is less

BACK STRENGTHENING

Extension

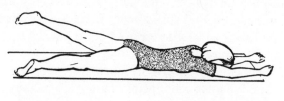

Beginning:
Lift one arm or one
leg at a time.

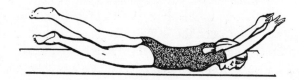

Intermediate:
Lift two
extremities at a time.

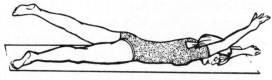

Advanced:
Lift all four
extremities at once.

Flexion

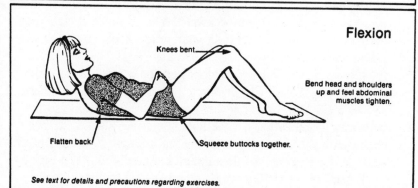

Knees bent

Bend head and shoulders
up and feel abdominal
muscles tighten.

Flatten back.

Squeeze buttocks together.

See text for details and precautions regarding exercises.

danger to your vertebrae if you do not bring your head and chest upright as you would doing a conventional sit-up. You may provide even further hedge against spinal injury if you keep a small pillow behind your back so your lower back is held in extension while your abdominal muscles tighten.

Fit people without osteoporosis maintain back flexion by touching their toes. You can more gently improve flexibility if you lie on your back and draw your knees up to your chest.

Another gentle way to improve back flexion is done sitting in a straight chair. Slowly bend forward and stretch your fingers to the floor alongside your feet. "Crawl" your fingers backward slowly, feeling the bend of each level of your spine. If you have osteoporosis, even these gentle exercises are some risk, but if you do them patiently it is not likely they will cause fracture.

Extension exercises stretch the front of the spine and do not pose the threat of compression fracture that flexion exercises do. Bending over backward from a standing position may cause you to fall. Back extension flexibility can be more safely done sitting. Bend forward at the hips, then arch your lower back and thrust head and shoulders backward. You can also stretch your back in extension if you lie on your stomach and prop yourself up on your elbows.

Lie on your stomach to do extension strengthening exercises. If you are already fit, stretch your arms over your head and then lift both arms and both legs at the same time so that only your abdomen touches the floor. Beginners should start with one arm and then one leg at a time; as strength is gained, progress to two extremities, then three, and finally four at a time.

Extension, flexibility, and strengthening exercises are pertinent to osteoporosis. Keeping joints free so your back will straighten and keeping muscles strong to pull your back straight helps you to stand tall. Extension exercises counteract the forward stooping, kyphotic posture that is both a cause and result of compression fracture.

Keep your back flexible for side-to-side bending. Fit people can stretch their hands down along the sides of their legs from a standing position. Those who must be more cautious with their spines and their balance should side-stretch while seated. Sit upright, lean back a little, and then bend directly to the side. Stretch your fingertips toward the floor first on one side of the chair, then on the other.

Hip Exercises: Strong hip muscles keep hipbones strong and help to prevent falls. One of the safest and most efficient hip and thigh muscle-strengthening exercises is the wall slide. Stand with your back flat against the wall and your heels away from the wall. Bend your hips and knees a little so you slide a few inches down the wall, then straighten your hips and knees so you slide back up the wall. Slowly increase the depth and duration of your bends. Do not underestimate how difficult this exercise can be. Start out very easily and progress slowly so that you do not get to a point from which you cannot rise safely.

Wall slides strengthen muscles in back of the hip (hip extensors) and front of the thigh (quadriceps). Muscles along the outside of the hip (abductors) are very important for strength, and those along the inside of the hip (adductors) are critical for balance and coordination.

From a sitting position, try to spread your knees against resistance that you supply with your hands along the outside of your knees. Then put your hand resistance along the insides of your knees and force your knees together. Straining against resistance to spread and close your knees will strengthen your hip abductors and adductors. Another good way to strengthen hip abductors is to lie on your side and lift your top leg, knee straight, directly toward the ceiling.

Leg Exercises: To strengthen your calf muscles, support yourself on a chairback and push your body weight up onto your tiptoes. Walk on your tiptoes and on your heels to strengthen your lower leg muscles and develop balance and coordination. If you are uncertain of your balance, hold on to someone or to a rail.

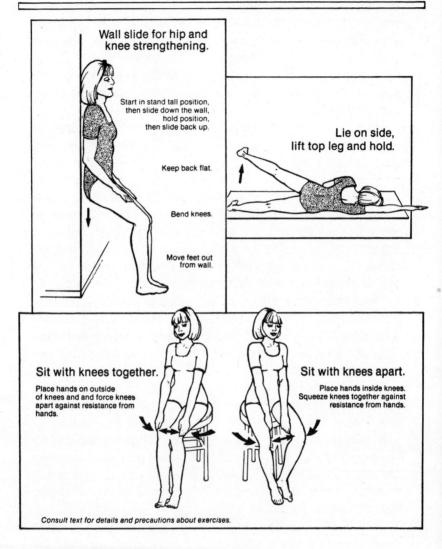

Wall slide for hip and knee strengthening.

Start in stand tall position, then slide down the wall, hold position, then slide back up.

Keep back flat.

Bend knees.

Move feet out from wall.

Lie on side, lift top leg and hold.

Sit with knees together.

Place hands on outside of knees and and force knees apart against resistance from hands.

Sit with knees apart.

Place hands inside knees. Squeeze knees together against resistance from hands.

Consult text for details and precautions about exercises.

Posture Exercise: At any time you do not have something else on your mind, you can practice the stand-tall exercise. Do it standing, sitting, or lying down. Tuck your chin in and raise your head so your neck gets longer. Pinch your shoulder blades in back so your arms roll back at the shoulders. Suck in your stomach and pinch your buttock muscles together so your lower back becomes flatter and longer. Imagine that there is a wire from the sky attached to the top of your head and that you are being pulled taller.

You cannot maintain the extreme position of standing tall all the time. However, you should strive to make your normal posture as near that as you can—and at least avoid the slumped opposite extreme.

Coordination: Most sports and ball games are good exercises in coordination. Dancing is good for balance. Aerobic dance routines combine exercises so that you get the diversity of movement that you miss in isolated strengthening and flexibility exercises. Square dancing, ballroom dancing, and other forms of social dancing are good for coordination. Walking on a beam is good hip exercise, but should be done with help standing by.

Endurance: When exercise is credited for benefits to heart, lungs, bowels, psyche, and general well-being, the reference is usually to endurance exercises. Endurance exercises must allow sustained elevated pulse and breathing rates. The participant cannot either stop for rest or become so exhausted that continuation is impossible. Such exercises are said to be "aerobic," which means that although oxygen is being burned at an increased rate, there is not a progressive oxygen deficit in the tissues, and the heart and lungs can keep up with the muscles' demands.

You must control the power and tempo of your efforts, or you will do too much or too little and not sustain a beneficial exercise level. Most sports and strengthening exercises require too much stop-and-go movement to be good for endurance. Aerobic dance is good for endurance if you do not stop to rest between the various exercises. Swimming, rowing, and bicycling are good endurance exercises if you do them properly. Rowing machines and stationary bicycles free you from concerns about weather, are safe, and are usually easy to sustain at a beneficial level. They may be the best endurance exercises for people who must limit the weight they bear on their legs, but the limited weight-bearing is a disadvantage to the prevention of osteoporosis. Bearing weight through your legs strengthens bones in your legs, hips, and spine. Walking or jogging provides the best combination of general fitness and osteoporosis protection.

There is no formula to tell you how much fitness and how much osteoporosis protection you get for each mile of walking or running. People who jog for forty-five minutes every other day stay very fit by cardiovascular standards, but we do not know if that applies to bones.

Long-distance runners have very dense bones, and sedentary people get osteoporosis. Somewhere in the middle ground there may be an answer to the question "How much is enough?" We do not know that answer; it is probably different for each individual. Certainly, what is safe and what is practical vary for each individual.

Jogging may be the best endurance exercise for people who are fit, but except for young and fit people, jogging is not a good beginning exercise. For many older or disabled people, jogging is not practical. For most people, walking is a good way to begin endurance exercise, and for many it is the best permanent exercise for endurance and bone strengthening.

You should begin endurance training by doing an amount of exercise that seems way too easy for you. Both good and bad effects of endurance training are cumulative. Foot, knee, and hip pains occur if you progress too rapidly. Such pains are usually caused by tendinitis or sore muscles; some of the worst pain comes from stress fractures. The injuries of overuse that cause such pains occur because of the accumulation of repeated minor injuries.

You may get by with slightly overdoing on one or two outings, but you will not if you repeat your efforts over several days.

If you begin with a very easy effort and experience no soreness from it, repeat the same effort over the next week. If you still experience no ill effects, increase your effort, but only by about 5 or 10 percent. If you had been walking 1.0 mile per day for a week and noticed no ill effects, then increase to no more than 1.1 mile per day for the next week. Do not try to increase daily, do not see how much you can do at one time, and do not increase your efforts by more than 10 percent each week. When you work up to a higher level of fitness, you will need to be even more cautious about increasing your weekly totals.

Begin a walking program by scheduling a time and a place to walk every day. Resolve to make your time for walking a permanent part of your life. Joggers can maintain fitness with workouts every other day, but those who walk for fitness do best if they schedule a time almost every day. Try to find a place where you can walk without interruption. City streets with traffic and stoplights are not good; neither are neighborhoods where you will be tempted to stop and talk. Sustained effort is essential for fitness.

Unfortunately, in the United States it is not always easy to find good places to walk. Caesar banned oxcarts from certain streets in Rome so people could walk, but few American cities have followed his example. If you cannot find good places to walk and wish to investigate and work toward solutions, write for information from the Walking Association, 3717 North 27 Street, Arlington VA 22207.

Make your time, find your place, then take your first walk— one short enough and slow enough that you know you will not feel exhausted or be sore afterward. Whether that is ten yards or three miles, accept what is a safe start for you and commit yourself to a slow, steady, patient progress. Each week, increase your distance by 5 or 10 percent.

Once you can walk three miles, you may wish to start increasing your speed. Time yourself at the pace you have been using for a few days. For the next week try to reduce your time by 5 percent or less. If you had been walking the distance in sixty minutes, try to cut it to fifty-seven minutes; or, if that proves too strenuous, cut it to fifty-nine minutes. Every week, walk the distance a little faster. When you are walking so fast that it would be more efficient to run, you are ready to begin jogging part of the way, if your goal is to jog.

Set goals based on your needs and abilities: you can always adjust your goals. Some people who never dreamed of running start jogging after they have become fit from walking and other exercises. Many people should not, and do not, ever jog a step but keep themselves fit and keep their bones strong by walking every day. How far and how fast you must walk to keep your bones strong are questions that current information does not answer. The best answer is that the more you walk at a brisk, uninterrupted pace, the better.

EXERCISE SUMMARY

You can choose from a great variety of exercises and fitness activities, but you must be sure certain ingredients are in your plans. First, you must be motivated; you must make a lifetime commitment to keep yourself fit. Second, you should have fun with your fitness program; include other people, and do not push yourself to exhaustion. Third, include each of the goals of endurance, strength, flexibility, posture, and coordination. Fourth, be patient; it takes three months or more of persistent effort before you see substantial results.

Start where you are. If you are confined to a chair, it is better to rock in a rocking chair than it is to sit still. Do not try to begin with your maximum effort and repeat that every day. Start easy and progress slowly. Do, however, be aggressive about finding help. Many schools, hospitals, and recreation centers offer supervised exercise programs for all age groups. Athletic organizations and health spas have exercise equipment and provide lessons or group sessions. If you cannot find an organization to provide what you need, find some other people with similar needs and form your own group.

Do not be discouraged by failure. Sometimes progress is unexplainably slow. Mistakes are easily made, so expect some times when you are sore or injured from overdoing. Rest for a while, then start up again on a less-demanding schedule. Seek help if you need it. Do not give up because of temporary setbacks: you have too much to gain.

Afterword

Parts of this book are hard to understand; some parts may even seem contradictory. I make no apology for that. Osteoporosis is not a simple subject. There are too many aspects and too many exceptions to reduce reliable information to a few paragraphs. Attempts to make osteoporosis seem simple may do a disservice and may even be dangerous.

Look back over the chapters to review the whole scope of the problem; then focus on the details most pertinent to you. The glossary and index that follow will help with unfamiliar words and subjects that may be hard to find.

MORE HELP

If you have read and understood this book, you know a great deal more than most people do about osteoporosis. You know more than many professionals do about the full scope of the problem. Most professionals deal with one or another special aspect of osteoporosis, rather than handling the full spectrum. Professionals may have very specialized knowledge about one aspect of osteoporosis and remain relatively uninformed about other aspects. Many gynecologists know a great deal about hormones and very little about fractures; the opposite is true for orthopedic surgeons.

Although you may know some things about osteoporosis that even the professionals do not, competent professionals provide you with a service that you simply cannot provide for yourself. The experiences of facing problems from osteoporosis with many different people over many years enable a qualified professional to bring to your case objectivity and experience that you cannot find in self-analysis.

The importance of osteoporosis has not received enough attention in our society. Medical and other professionals have not been immune to the inappropriate lack of attention to osteoporosis. Therefore, you cannot assume that otherwise perfectly competent and well-meaning physicians will aggressively advise you about osteoporosis. So while you need your physician's help, you may have to ask for it. Do not reject your physician because of that or because he or she may not know about some aspect of osteoporosis. The medical community and their patients must learn about osteoporosis together, and they need each other.

If your doctor does not seem to know or care enough about osteoporosis, talk to him or her about it and ask to be referred to someone who does. If your doctor disagrees with something you may have decided from your self-analysis, you may want to ask for another opinion about that; but remember to respect your doctor's judgment, because he or she has a perspective that you cannot obtain from self-analysis.

Your family-practice physician or internist should be the first one you consult about osteoporosis, or at least should know about your concerns and what you are doing about it. Gynecologists and endocrinologists are specialists with expert knowledge regarding hormone treatments. Orthopedic surgeons specialize in fracture care and rehabilitation. Individual doctors in any of those specialties may have a particular interest in osteoporosis and may provide care for aspects of osteoporosis outside the usual scope of their specialties. If you think a specialist you are seeing may not have an interest in the full scope of osteoporosis problems, make the physician aware of your concerns. He or she should either be able to reassure you of his or her competence and interest or should be able to suggest others for you to consult.

The information about physicians applies to osteopaths. Osteopathic physicians are governed by requirements similar to those of medical doctors. Osteopathic medicine once relied upon spinal manipulation as treatment for a wide range of medical disorders. However, modern osteopaths may specialize just as medical doctors do. The word "osteopath" does not imply any special knowledge about bone disorders such as osteoporosis. If your physician is an osteopath, you cannot assume that he or she knows any more or less about osteoporosis than a medical doctor.

Many nonphysicians participate in the professional care of osteoporosis problems. Rehabilitation from fractures often requires the special skills of a physical therapist and/or an occupational therapist. Nurses and social workers often contribute to the care of people whose injuries bring them to the hospital. Dietitians provide reliable information about the nutritional aspects of osteoporosis care. Pharmacists give advice about medication and diet supplement ingredients, and can help interpret the labels on over-the-counter drugs. All of these professionals, who have degrees, must be registered. If you doubt whether someone you have consulted is qualified to advise you, ask your doctor or the hospital administrator to check on it for you.

Many people with marginal qualifications advertise willingness to advise and care for problems related to osteoporosis. The specialists mentioned previously should either be well qualified or at least aware of their limitations. Some chiropractors, nutritionists, and other health-care advisers are not really qualified to give advice about an issue as complex as osteoporosis. They may be able to provide some specialized help, but you should check any information from such sources with your physician.

Many chiropractors aggressively solicit patients with back pain. Some chiropractors are aware of the special problems of osteoporosis and provide their patients with solid information about nutrition, exercise, and appropriate consultation, but many do not. Vigorous chiropractic manipulation of an osteoporotic spine can cause fracture. If osteoporosis is the problem, chiropractic treatments can be useless and expensive, and needlessly delay important treatment. If you are being treated by a chiropractor, make sure the advice you have been given is consistent with what you have read in this book and what you have been told by your physician.

HOPE

This book gives many answers to questions about osteoporosis. The answers we can give now are much better than the ones we used to give. Still, many of our answers are indefinite and qualified. We do not know enough yet—but the interest is growing, and research is bringing us better answers every year.

Fluoridation of water has reduced tooth decay by 30 percent in ten years. Will we see a reduction in osteoporosis because of fluoridation? Will we find doses and ways to give fluoride or other elements that will prevent osteoporosis? Will we come to understand the chemistry of the bone-building cells so we can energize them to work better? Will we understand the coupling mechanism better so we can stimulate the formation of new bone and simultaneously retard the resorption of old bone? Will we better understand the chemistry of why estrogens and vitamin D are important to bone? Probably so. Good research is progressing along those and many other lines. As the public becomes more interested in osteoporosis, better answers will come from research.

SPREADING THE WORD

Millions of people have osteoporosis; millions more are well on their way to developing osteoporosis and do not know it. Most of the fractures from osteoporosis could be prevented if people just knew and practiced preventives available right now; if we merely delayed the progress of osteoporosis by five years, we would prevent nearly half the fractures.

Osteoporosis prevention begins in the embryo with good prenatal care, continues through childhood when we build the size and strength of our bones, continues throughout adult life when nutrition and exercise maintain our bone strengths, becomes critical at the time of menopause when sudden losses of bone may occur from hormone deficits, and is especially important in old age when fractures threaten and good nutrition and exercise practices become even more difficult. All ages have an interest in osteoporosis.

In spite of the widespread need for information about osteoporosis, little is available to the general public. I tried to assemble all the information that I thought was pertinent and reliable for this book. *Stand Tall* by Morris Notelovitz, M.D., and Marsha Ware (Triad Publishing Co., Gainesville, Florida, 1982) is another good book about osteoporosis, with special emphasis on hormones and diet. A free, but brief, pamphlet is available from the NIH (write for "Osteoporosis: Cause, Treatment, Prevention," NIH Publication 83-2226, prepared by the National Institute of Arthritis, Diabetes, and Digestive and Kidney Diseases and published by the U.S. Department of Health and Human Services, Public Health Service, National Institutes of Health, Bethesda, Ma !and 20205).

"Osteoporosis" is a difficult word, unfamiliar to most people. It sounds dreadfully medical and scientific. We are, however, stuck with it. Neither the medical community nor the general public is going to begin calling this problem by some less-imposing name. We need to accept the word osteoporosis and use it around our children, our parents, and our friends until the strangeness of it wears off. We need to use the word osteoporosis until everyone is familiar with the word and familiar with all the trouble that lurks behind the meaning of the word. We need to use it until teachers teach about osteoporosis in grade schools; until teenagers understand the relationship between the fast food they eat and the way Grandma's back is bent over; until chairpersons of women's club programs include osteoporosis on their list of topics for discussion; until doctors become aware that every patient wants to know what he or she can do to prevent osteoporosis; and until older people aggressively pursue programs that help them prevent and overcome the complications of osteoporosis.

Having read this book, you now know a great deal about osteoporosis. You have two responsibilities. The first is to do all you can to keep yourself from suffering from osteoporosis. The second is to spread the word.

Glossary

Abduction Movement away from the center of the body, as in spreading the legs apart.

Abductors Muscles that pull the limbs away from the center of the body, such as those from the pelvis to the thigh, along the side of the hip.

Absorptiometry Bone density measurement that depends upon the bone's absorption of different X-ray dosages.

Acetabulum Portion of the pelvis that forms the pelvic side of the hip joint; socket of the ball-and-socket hip joint.

Adrenal glands Glands that sit atop each kidney; produce adrenaline and cortisone-like hormones.

Adrenaline Hormone produced by the adrenal glands; increases heart rate, blood pressure, and metabolic rate.

Adrenopause Period of life when the adrenal glands begin to decrease the amount of hormones they produce; usually after age sixty.

Aerobic exercise Exercise that can be sustained without breathlessness and progressive deficit of oxygen.

Alkaline phosphatase An enzyme that is important in both bone and liver metabolism.

Alzheimer's disease A brain disease characterized by impairment of memory and other intellectual functions.

Amino acids Nitrogen-containing molecules that are the building blocks of protein.

Anabolic Body-building; constructive metabolism; tending to increase body mass.

Anabolic steroids Hormones or chemically similar drugs that may contribute to the strengthening of muscle and bone.

Androgen A hormone that produces masculine characteristics in the human body.

Angulated fracture A broken bone in which the pieces no longer maintain their normal alignment, forming an abnormal angle at the fracture site.

Anorexia nervosa Psychological inability to eat; leads to the effects of starvation.

Antacids Medicines that neutralize stomach acid.

Anterior Toward the front; opposite of **posterior.**

Arthritis Inflammation of a joint or joints.

Ascorbate The salt of the six-carbon organic acid ascorbic acid. *See also* **Vitamin C.**

Aseptic necrosis *See* **Avascular necrosis.**

Atresia A process of withering and shrinking with age; usually refers to the fate of unexpelled ova in the ovaries.

Austin Moore prosthesis One type of metal replacement for the head of the femur; supported by a stem that fits into the canal of the femur.

Avascular necrosis Death of a bone or portion of a bone due to loss of its blood supply. Also called **aseptic necrosis.**

Bimalleolar fracture Broken ankle; fracture through both the lateral malleolus of the fibula and medial malleolus of the tibia at the ankle.

Binder Soft, elastic band used to wrap around the abdomen and lower back or around the chest; provides back support and comfort.

Biopsy Surgical procedure in which tissue is removed for the purpose of diagnostic examination.

Body of vertebra Block-shaped portion of the vertebra; located at the front of the spine. Also called **centrum.**

Bone mass Substance of bone; for practical purposes, equivalent to the weight of bone.

Bone personality Characteristics of one's bone that are unique to him or her.

Bone scan Map of bone activity obtained by injection of a radioisotope. Also called **scintimetry.**

Brace A more or less rigid support usually made from plastics or steel; more substantial and confining than a binder or corset.

Calcitonin A hormone produced by specialized cells in the thyroid gland; acts to conserve calcium in bone.

Calcium A metal element found abundantly in nature, especially in bones and shells.

Calcium bank The storage of calcium held in one's bones.

Calcium blocker Medicine used to regulate heart and blood vessel function; also called **channel blocker.**

Calcium hydroxyapatite crystals Crystals composed primarily of calcium, hydrogen, oxygen, and phosphorus; basic type of crystal found in bone.

Caliper Mechanical device used for precise measurement of linear distance.

Callus Living tissue that forms around a broken bone, usually leading to healing of the fracture.

Capsule (of joint) Collagen fibers forming a ligament that encloses a joint.

Carbonates Salts of carbonic acid; calcium carbonate, for example.

Carbonic acid An organic acid containing one carbon atom.

Carotid pulse Pulsation of the carotid artery, located on each side and toward the front of the neck.

Carpal tunnel syndrome Pain and/or numbness of the hand due to pressure on the median nerve at the wrist.

CAT (CT) scan (computerized axial tomography) Computer-assisted X-ray technique for providing images in various planes.

Center of gravity Center of body weight; the axis about which a suspended body would rotate.

Centrum *See* **Body of vertebra.**

Cervix Lowest portion of the uterus; mouth of the womb.

Channel blocker *See* **Calcium blocker.**

Chiropractor Practitioner of a discipline based on the theory that many symptoms are explained by malalignment of the spine; not a medical doctor.

Cholecalciferol   Chemical name of the form of vitamin D obtained from animal sources.

Cholelithiasis   Gallstones; presence of stones in the gallbladder or bile ducts.

Cholesterol   A fat substance present in high concentrations in red meats, eggs, butter fat, and other foods; diets high in cholesterol may cause fat deposits in arteries.

Climacteric   Period of life when critical changes occur; usually refers to the menopause in women.

Closed fracture   Broken bone that is not open to the outside, not broken through the skin; opposite of **open fracture.**

Closed reduction   Replacement, or setting, of broken bones into satisfactory position and alignment without performing an open operation.

Codfish vertebra   Collapse of the body of a vertebra in such a way that the X-ray picture forms a silhouette similar to that of a codfish.

Collagen   Protein that is the major nonmineral component of bone; also the major component of tendons, ligaments, and scars.

Colles' fracture   Broken radius at the wrist, usually with displacement of the distal bone fragment dorsal to the long axis of the forearm.

Comminuted fracture   Bone broken into more than two pieces.

Complete fracture   Bone broken so that the fracture line extends through the whole circumference of the bone.

Composite beam   A support structure composed of two or more dissimilar materials.

Compound fracture   *See* **Open fracture.**

Compression fracture   Bone broken by crushing the bone together; most often refers to crushing fractures of bodies of vertebrae.

Compton scatter   A property of radiation that can be used to measure bone density.

Computerized axial tomography   *See* **CAT scan.**

Condyles   Rounded ends of long bones that form joint surfaces; refers especially to the ends of the humerus at the elbow and the femur at the knee.

Conjugated estrogens   A blended composition of different naturally occurring estrogens.

Corpus luteum   Structure in the ovary, derived from the follicle after ovulation; produces progesterone.

Corset   Support device worn around the waist and lower chest.

Cortex   Outer shell of bone; hard, compact outer portion of a bone.

Cortical bone   Densely packed bone that makes up the bone's cortex.

Corticosteroids   A group of steroid hormones produced by the outer portion of the adrenal gland, or chemically derived drugs that have similar structures and effects; includes cortisone. *See also* **Steroids.**

Cortisone   One of the steroid hormones formed by the adrenal glands. Other steroids and drugs that produce similar effects are sometimes imprecisely called cortisone. *See also* **Corticosteroids; Glucocorticoids.**

Coupling   Linked functions; with reference to bone, the linkage of bone resorption to bone formation.

CPR (cardiopulmonary resuscitation)   Technique for emergency revival of someone whose heartbeat or breathing has stopped.

Crush fracture   Breaking of a bone by crushing the cortical surfaces together; usually refers to such fractures in bodies of vertebrae.

Cushing's syndrome   Effects of excessive cortisone; includes high blood pressure, high blood sugar, osteoporosis, and changes in appearance.

Delayed union   A fracture that has not healed within the predicted time but has healed or still may heal.

Densitometer   Machine for measurement of bone density.

Density   Mass per unit volume. In bone, density is proportional to the weight of solid bone in a given volume of bone.

Diabetes   Disease characterized by high blood sugar and deficiency of insulin.

Dietitian   Professional who provides advice about diet and nutrition. Qualified professionals may display the initials R.D., meaning Registered Dietitian.

Disc (intervertebral disc)   Joint between bodies of vertebrae; composed of a circular ligament, the anulus fibrosus, and a gel-like center, the nucleus pulposus.

Displaced fracture   Broken bone in which the fragments have separated from one another at the fracture site.

Distal   Away from the center of the body; opposite of **proximal.**

Distraction   Pulling apart; separating by pulling in opposite directions.

Disuse osteoporosis   Loss of bone mass because of insufficient stress to the bone, as might occur from lack of use.

Diuretics   Chemicals that increase the amount of urine produced by the kidneys.

Diurnal rhythms   Cyclic changes in body function that occur approximately daily.

Dorsal   Thoracic or chest area. Also, may designate direction, in which case it means nearly the same as **posterior;** toward the back side of the trunk or an extremity.

Dorsal spine   Thoracic or chest portion of the spine.

Dowager's hump   Rounded prominence of the upper spine, common in older women with osteoporosis.

Dual photon absorptiometry   Bone density test done by passing beams from two different radioactive sources through the bone.

Endocrine glands   Hormone-producing glandular structures scattered throughout the body.

Endocrinologist   Medical doctor who specializes in management of disorders of the endocrine glands.

Endocrinology   Study of hormones and endocrine glands.

Endometrium   Inner lining layer of the uterus.

Endosteum   Inside surface layer of bone.

Epiphyseal growth plate   Growth sites near the ends of long bones.

Epiphysis (plural, **epiphyses**)   End of a long bone; portion of a long bone that participates in a joint.

Ergocalciferol   Chemical name of the form of vitamin D found in plants.

Estradiol   Chemical name of a type of estrogen hormone; the main estrogen produced by the ovary.

Estrogens   A group of hormones produced by the ovaries and adrenal glands; essential to the reproductive functions of women.

Estrones   Chemical name of a type of estrogen hormone; the main form of estrogens produced by the adrenal glands.

Extension   Stretched out straight; sometimes means beyond straight; for example, arching the lower back so as to look at the ceiling is called extension of the back.

Extensor muscles   Muscles that produce extension; sometimes used to refer specifically to muscles that extend the back, but can refer to any other muscles that act to extend a joint.

Facet joints   Joints where adjacent vertebrae join at the back of the spine.

Fallopian tubes   Tube-shaped tissue from the ovaries to the uterus; passageways for ova.

Femur   Thighbone.

Fibers   *See* **Fibrils.**

Fibrils   Fine strands of collagen or other protein; may be woven together to form fibers, which are larger strands.

Fibrous union   Healing of a fracture by soft-tissue scar, as opposed to bony union.

Fibula   Long bone along the outside of the leg; smaller of the two bones that span from the knee to the ankle.

Flat bones   Bones that are more or less flat and lack tubular structure, such as the skull, shoulder blade, and pelvis.

Flexion   Motion toward a bent, or flexed, position. Opposite of **extension.**

Flexor muscles   Muscles that move joints into flexion; with regard to the spine, refers to abdominal muscles that bend the body forward.

Fluoride   The negatively charged ion of fluorine; forms compounds that can be taken internally to strengthen teeth and, in some cases, bones.

Fluorine   An element which, in its pure form, usually exists as a gas.

Follicle (ovarian)   Cells and fluid that surround and nourish an ovum prior to ovulation.

Fracture   A break in the normal structure of bone.

FSH (follicle-stimulating hormone)   Hormone produced by the pituitary gland; stimulates the development of a follicle.

Galactorrhea   Abnormal discharge of milk from the breasts.

GH (growth hormone)   Hormone produced by the pituitary gland; stimulates growth.

Glucocorticoids   Glucose-elevating hormones from the adrenal glands; includes cortisone and similar substances. See **Corticosteroids; Cortisone.**

Gluconate   Salt of the six-carbon organic acid gluconic acid; for example, calcium gluconate.

Greater trochanter (of femur)   Knob of bone at the outer, upper end of the thighbone; site of insertion of muscles that abduct and extend the hip.

Greenstick fracture   Break through one cortex of a bone with bending of the adjacent cortex; bone broken in the way a green stick breaks.

Gynecologist   Medical doctor who specializes in the care of the reproductive organs of women.

Haversian canals   Small canals that pass through compact, cortical bone.

Haversian surface   Surface of the small passageways through cortical bone.

HDL (high-density lipoprotein)   One blood component of fat/protein molecules; higher levels of HDL correlate with fewer fat deposits in arteries, as opposed to **LDL** and **VLDL.**

Head (of radius, humerus, femur)   Rounded ends of bones such as the radius at the elbow, humerus at the shoulder, and femur at the hip.

Histochemistry   Tests that combine microscopic analysis with chemical staining techniques.

Hormone   Natural, blood-borne substances that regulate various body functions.

Hot flush (hot flash)   Symptoms of being too hot that are not explained by activity or environmental temperature; usually associated with menopause.

Humerus   Bone of the upper arm; spans from shoulder to elbow.

Hydroxyproline   An amino acid that is a characteristic component of the nonmineral portion of bone.

Hyperparathyroidism   Effects of excessive activity of parathyroid hormone, one of which may be osteoporosis.

Hypertension   High blood pressure.

Hyperthyroidism   Effects of excessive activity of thyroid hormone, one of which may be osteoporosis.

Hysterectomy   Surgical removal of the uterus. Total or complete hysterectomy usually means surgical removal of the ovaries and fallopian tubes as well as the uterus.

Idiopathic Of unknown cause.

Idiopathic osteoporosis Osteoporosis that is not related to some known, specific, underlying disease.

Ilium Largest bone of the pelvis; bone felt at the waist.

Impacted fracture Broken bone in which one broken piece is pushed into the other, similar to the way a ball of ice cream is pushed down onto a cone.

Incomplete fracture Broken bone in which the fracture does not extend through the whole circumference of the bone.

Innominate bone Combination of the three bones which, in the adult, fuse together to form each side of the pelvis.

Insulin Hormone produced by the pancreas; promotes entry of glucose into cells.

Internal fixation Surgical placement of devices to hold bones together, usually metal devices used to hold together fractured pieces of bone.

Inter-trochanteric (I.T.) Line or area between the greater trochanter and the lesser trochanter at the upper end of the femur. *See also* **Trochanteric.**

Intervertebral disc *See* **Disc.**

Intra-articular fracture Broken bone in which one or more of the fracture lines extend into a joint surface.

Ions Charged combining forms of atoms or groups of atoms.

Ischium Posterior and lower bones of the pelvis; bones of the greatest contact pressure when sitting.

Isotopes Atoms of the same element that contain different numbers of neutrons but the same number of protons; different isotopes of the same element have similar chemical properties but different degrees of stability.

Isotretinoin (Accutane) Drug derived from vitamin A, used for the treatment of acne.

I.U. (international units) Dosages based on weight or activity of a drug; usually an arbitrary unit agreed upon by scientists to provide uniform understanding.

Kidney stones Accumulations of solid material in the kidneys or urinary tract; may or may not contain calcium.

Knowles pin A type of threaded metal pin used to hold together fractures of the neck of the femur.

Kyphosis Backward pointing curve of the spine; up to about forty-five degrees is normal in the dorsal spine.

Lactase An enzyme from the intestine that aids digestion of lactose in milk.

Lactate Salt of the three-carbon organic acid, lactic acid.

Lactose A double sugar composed of glucose and galactose, present in milk.

Lateral To the side or from the side; opposite of **medial.**

LDL (low-density lipoprotein) One blood component of fat/protein molecules; high levels of LDL are correlated with increased deposits of fat in blood vessels. *See also* **HDL; VLDL.**

Lesser trochanter Knob of bone on the inside of the upper femur; site of insertion of muscles that flex the hip.

LH (luteinizing hormone) Hormone produced by the pituitary gland; stimulates ovulation.

Ligament Supporting structure from one bone to another; composed of fibers.

Ligamentum teres Ligament from the center of the acetabulum to the center of the head of the femur; inside the hip joint.

Lipoprotein Molecule formed by combination of fat and protein components.

Long bones Bones that are relatively long and tubular.

Lordosis Forward-pointing curvature of the spine; some lordosis is normal in the cervical and lumbar spines.

Lumbar Region of the back between the lowest ribs and the pelvis.

Lumbar spine Portion of the spine between the thoracic spine and pelvis; composed of five lumbar vertebrae and their attachments.

Madder Plant from which a red dye is derived; important in the history of the understanding of bone growth.

Magnesium Metal element present in small amounts in bone, muscle, and other tissues.

Malleolus Knob at the end of a bone; the lateral malleolus of the fibula and medial malleolus of the tibia form the side walls of the ankle joint.

Marrow space Space inside bone; bound by trabeculae of bone; contains bone marrow cells.

Mature union Broken bone healed by strong, reformed bone across the previous fracture site.

MDR (minimum daily requirement) Amount of a nutrient below which symptoms or effects of disease would occur.

Medial Toward the midline of the body; opposite of **lateral.**

Median nerve Large nerve in the arm and hand; passes through the carpal tunnel at the wrist.

Menopause Time of hormonal changes in women when menstruation and reproductive functions diminish, then cease.

Microfractures Tiny cracks in portions of a bone, usually discernible only with a microscope or other special testing.

Milieu Environment, surroundings.

Mineral An inorganic substance having a consistent set of physical properties and a specific chemical formula; not derived from animal or vegetable sources.

Mineralization Process by which minerals are deposited on or within nonmineral tissue; for example, deposition of calcium crystals on collagen in bone.

Mobilization Creation of movement. May refer to chemical events leading to movement of minerals out of bone. May also refer to physical events such as the movement of joints.

Multiple myeloma A form of bone-marrow cancer. Sometimes called **Myeloma.**

Multivitamins Combinations of three or more vitamins into a common preparation.

Myeloma *See* **Multiple myeloma.**

Nails (orthopedic) Relatively large, metal appliances inserted by surgeons to hold together broken bones.

Neck (of femur, humerus, or radius) Portion of a long bone that connects the main, shaft portion of the bone to the head of the bone.

Neutron activation A technique of measuring the total amount of calcium in the body.

Nonunion Site of a broken bone that has never healed, bone to bone, and is past the time when such healing could be reasonably expected to occur.

Nutritionist   Anyone who claims to be an expert on nutrition or diet; does not imply any special qualifications.

Occupational therapist   A professional trained in rehabilitative measures designed to qualify a sick or injured person for productive activity; also expert in use of assistive devices.

Oculo-manual syndrome   Excessive attention to and overprotection of an injured wrist or hand.

Olecranon   Upper end of the ulna; forms the bone prominence at the back of the elbow.

Oophorectomy   Surgical removal of the ovaries.

Open fracture   Broken bone with an injury to the skin and soft tissues so that the fracture site has been exposed to the outside. Sometimes called **compound fracture.**

Open reduction   Surgical operation for replacement of broken pieces of bone into their proper relationships to one another.

Organic acids   Carbon-containing molecules that give up hydrogen ions in solution; contain the atomic configuration -COOH.

Organic salts   The combination of an organic acid with a positively charged ion to form a salt, such as calcium carbonate.

ORIF (open reduction, internal fixation)   Open reduction, combined with insertion of devices to hold together the broken pieces.

Orthopedic surgeon   Medical doctor trained to practice orthopedic surgery. Also called *orthopedist.*

Orthopedic surgery   Medical specialty that includes diagnosis and treatment, including surgery, for disorders of the spine, arms, and legs; includes care of broken bones.

Osteoarthritis   Most common of the inflammatory disorders of joints; sometimes called wear-and-tear, or degenerative, arthritis.

Osteoblasts   Bone cells that produce new bone.

Osteoclasts   Bone cells that resorb bone.

Osteocytes   Bone cells that maintain bone.

Osteogenesis imperfecta   Inherited disease that results in weak, easily broken bones.

Osteomalacia   Disease characterized by inadequate deposition of calcium and other minerals in bone.

Osteopath Medical practitioner who possesses the degree D.O. (Doctor of Osteopathy).

Osteopathy Medical practice of osteopaths; once based upon spinal manipulation, has now evolved to embrace principles essentially the same as those of medical doctors.

Osteopenia Decreased mass of bone; a nonspecific term that may encompass decreased bone mass of any cause.

Osteophyte Localized enlargement of bone, usually at the site of ligament insertion. Sometimes called *spur*.

Osteoporosis A primary disease of multiple causes or a bone disorder secondary to any of several known causes, the common characteristics being decreased bone mass and increased susceptibility to fracture.

Ovaries Female reproductive organs; contain ova; produce estrogen and progestogen hormones.

Overuse osteoporosis Osteoporosis related to excessive physical stress; an uncommon phenomenon observed in a few people undergoing extreme physical stress.

Ovulation Expulsion of an ovum from an ovary.

Ovum (plural, **ova**) Egg; female contribution to a new organism.

Oxalates Organic salts that may form kidney stones; in the intestines may decrease the absorption of calcium.

Parathormone *See* **Parathyroid hormone.**

Parathyroid glands Small glands located in the front of the neck; produce parathyroid hormone.

Parathyroid hormone (PTH, parathormone) Hormone produced by the parathyroid gland; important to calcium balance in blood, bone, and urine.

Patella Bone of the kneecap; a sesamoid bone within the tendon of the quadriceps muscle.

Perimenopausal Around the time of the menopause.

Periodontal Around the teeth; referring to the gingiva (gums).

Periosteum Outside lining layer of bone.

Personality (of bone) *See* **Bone personality.**

Phosphate Ion formed by a combination of phosphorus and oxygen.

Phosphorus Metal element that so readily combines with oxygen it seldom occurs in its pure form; a major component of bone mineral.

Photodensitometry   A test of bone density; measurement of the radiation absorbed by a bone from a beam directed from a radioactive source. Also called **photon absorptiometry.**

Photon absorptiometry   *See* **Photodensitometry.**

Physical therapist   Professional who administers physical treatment and exercise measures and guides physical rehabilitation.

Phytates   Organic compounds present in many foods; may impair calcium absorption.

Piezoelectric effect   An electric current induced by bending a crystal-containing substance.

Pinning (fracture)   Surgical insertion of metal wires or screwlike devices for the purpose of holding together broken pieces of bone.

Pituitary gland   Endocrine gland at the base of the brain; produces hormones that influence the activities of other endocrine glands.

Plafond (of tibia)   Ceiling; flat undersurface of the end of the tibia.

Plateau (of tibia)   High flat area; flat surfaces at the top of the tibia.

Polypeptides   Complex nitrogen-containing organic molecules; components of proteins.

Posterior   Toward the back; opposite of **anterior.**

Postmenopausal   After the menopause; after menstrual periods cease and estrogen production diminishes.

Pott's fracture   Fractures of the ankle, including fractures of both medial and lateral malleoli.

Premenopausal   Before any symptoms of menopause have occurred.

Prenatal vitamins   Vitamin and mineral combinations recommended for pregnant women.

Progesterone   Hormone produced by the corpus luteum of the ovary; stimulates the lining of the uterus to support a pregnancy.

Progestin   Naturally occurring or synthetically produced compound with effects and chemical structure similar to those of progesterone.

Progestogen   Compound with effects similar to those of progesterone. Sometimes used to distinguish compounds (derived from molecules somewhat chemically dissimilar to progesterone but having progesterone-like effects) from progestins, but often used, as in the text of this book, as a general term that refers to all natural and synthetic compounds with progesterone-like action.

Prolactin (PRL)   Hormone produced by the pituitary; helps initiate and sustain flow of milk from the breasts.

Prolactinoma Tumor of the prolactin-producing cells of the pituitary gland.

Prosthesis Artificial part, either external such as an artificial leg, or internal such as a metallic replacement of the head of the femur.

Proximal Relatively nearer to the center of the body; opposite of **distal.**

PTH *See* **Parathyroid hormone.**

Pubis The lower, front bone of each side of the pelvis; the two pubi join together in the anterior midline.

Quad cane Cane with four-legged platform to provide stable contact with the floor.

Quadriceps Muscles of the front of the thigh.

Radiographic absorptiometry *See* **Absorptiometry.**

Radiography Production of X-ray pictures.

Radius One of the two bones of the forearm; forms most of the bone surface on the near side of the wrist.

RDA (recommended daily allowance) The amount of a nutrient that should be present in the diet to ensure maintenance of adequate levels of that nutrient, as recommended by boards of scientists.

Receptor Receiving site; locations in living tissue where specific circulating molecules attach.

Reduce (fracture) Replace broken pieces of bone into more acceptable positions. Sometimes called *set.*

Remodeling (of bone) Natural process whereby a growing or healing bone is reshaped to the normal adult shape.

Resorption Process by which portions of bone are dissolved and carried away.

Respiratory acidosis The presence of excess acid in the blood because carbon dioxide has not been adequately removed by the lungs.

Rheumatoid arthritis A disease that may cause chronic inflammation of joints; may be destructive to joints. Sometimes called *crippling arthritis.*

Rheumatologist Physician who specializes in the diagnosis and nonsurgical care of joint diseases.

Rheumatology Medical specialty that deals with diagnosis and treatment of joint diseases and inflammatory diseases that may include joint symptoms.

Rickets Childhood bone disease caused by deficiency of vitamin D, either from dietary deficiency or from inborn error of vitamin-D metabolism.

Sacroiliac joint Site on each side of the pelvis where the sacrum joins the back of the iliac portion of the pelvis.

Sacrum Large bone at the base of the spine; solid base at the lower end of the spine; portion of the spine that joins the pelvis.

Salpingo-oophorectomy Surgical removal of the ovaries and fallopian tubes.

Saturated fats Fats that have their sites for hydrogen ions occupied; saturated fats cause more fat deposits in arteries than unsaturated fats.

Scan Test in which whole organs or body parts are measured or pictured for diagnostic purposes. *See* **Bone scan; CAT scan.**

Scintimetry *See* **Bone scan.**

Scoliosis Side-to-side curvature of the spine.

Scurvy Disease caused by deficiency of vitamin C.

Sesamoids Bones located within tendons.

Sex hormones Hormones produced by testes, ovaries, and adrenals that influence sexual functions.

Shaft Middle, tubular portion of a long bone.

Short bones Relatively small bones, of various shapes, such as the bones of the hands and feet.

Side plate Metal bar with screw holes in it; usually refers to the part of a device that attaches to the shaft of the femur to hold the pieces of a broken hip.

Sodium Metal element present in high concentration in most body tissues, but in relatively low concentration in bone.

Sodium fluoride Molecule composed of sodium and fluoride ions; a commonly available source of fluoride supplement.

Spinal cord Nerve cells and nerve tracts that extend from the brain to the end of the thoracic spine; relays and coordinates messages between the brain and peripheral nerves.

Spine Column of bones and attachments from the head to the pelvis, through which pass the spinal cord and spinal nerves.

Steroids A group of chemically similar organic compounds produced by the adrenal glands, ovaries, and testes, or chemically derived drugs with similar structures and effects. *See also* **Anabolic steroids; Corticosteroids; Cortisone; Glucocorticoids; Testosterone.**

Stones Solid accumulation of material in sites of fluid flow, such as in urinary tracts, bile tracts, and salivary ducts.

Stress fracture Break in a bone caused by repeated stresses that produce tiny cracks faster than the bone can repair them.

Stress riser Site where stresses concentrate.

Styloid (ulnar, radial) Pointed tip at the end of a bone; the radius and ulna both have styloid processes at the wrist.

Subtrochanteric fracture Break in the upper femur just below the level of the greater and lesser trochanters.

Supracondylar Area of bone just above the condyles, usually refers to the humerus above the elbow or the femur above the knee.

Sympathetic dystrophy Reaction to injury characterized by unusual degree and duration of pain and stiffness.

Technetium Radioactive element often used for bone scans.

Temperomandibular joint Joint where the jaw connects to the skull.

Tendinitis Inflammation of a tendon or tendon insertion.

Testosterone Steroid hormone produced by the testes and in lesser amounts by the ovaries and adrenals; creates masculine effects; male sex hormone.

Tetracycline An antibiotic used for the treatment and prevention of infections.

Thompson prosthesis One type of metal replacement for the head of the femur.

Thoracic Chest area.

Thoracic spine Portion of the spine between the neck and the lumbar spine; chest portion of the spine. Also called **dorsal spine.**

Thoracolumbar junction Lowest portion of the thoracic and upper portion of the lumbar spine; area where the thoracic and lumbar spines join.

Thrombophlebitis Inflammation of a vein with a blood clot in the vein.

Thyroid gland Gland in the front of the neck; produces thyroid hormone and calcitonin.

Thyroid hormone   Hormone produced by the thyroid gland; important regulator of metabolic rates.

Tibia   Large bone of the lower leg; spans from the knee to the ankle.

Total hip replacement   Operation to replace both the head of the femur and the surface of the acetabulum.

Trabecula (plural, **trabeculae**)   Support beam of bone; forms the interior structure of bone.

Trabecular bone   Portion of bone composed of the relatively loosely spaced interior beams of bone; as opposed to the dense, compact, exterior surface, which is called **cortical bone.**

Trace elements   Elements present in the body in very small amounts.

Traction   A pulling force, usually along the long axis of an extremity or of the body.

Trigintal rhythms   Changes that occur in approximately monthly cycles.

Trimalleolar fracture   Ankle fracture in which the lateral malleolus of the fibula and medial and posterior malleoli of the tibia are broken.

Trochanter   Large knob of bone to which tendons attach; usually refers to the greater and lesser trochanters of the upper femur.

Trochanteric   In the region of the trochanters of the upper femur. *See also* **Inter-trochanteric.**

Ulna   One of the two long bones of the forearm; larger at the elbow and smaller at the wrist.

Ultrasound   Sound waves above the audible frequency; used in medical diagnostics and treatment.

Undisplaced fracture   Broken bone in which the broken pieces remain in their normal positions and relationships to one another.

Union (of a fracture)   Healing of a broken bone.

Uric acid stones   Stones composed of uric acid salts; sometimes called *urate stones.*

Uterus   Female reproductive organ; site of growth of the embryo; womb.

Vertebra   One of the bones of the spine.

Vertebral body   *See* **Body of vertebra.**

Vitamin   Substance that is essential in small amounts in the diet to maintain good health.

Vitamin A A fat-soluble vitamin; supplements taken in excessive amounts can cause serious illness, including osteoporosis.

Vitamin C (ascorbic acid) A water-soluble vitamin; occurs in citrus fruits; deficiency causes scurvy.

Vitamin D A fat-soluble vitamin; deficiencies cause rickets in children and osteomalacia in adults.

VLDL (very low-density lipoproteins) Fat/protein blood component similar to LDL. *See* **LDL.**

Walker Four-legged device to assist walking; permits taking some weight and balance with both hands.

Wall slide Exercise done by bending the knees and hips while the back is supported against a wall.

Wedge fracture Fracture of the body of a vertebra; the front of the body is crushed down further than the back, leaving the body wedge-shaped.

Window (medicine dosage) The dose range of medicine between the lowest effective dose and the highest safe dose.

Withdrawal bleeding Vaginal bleeding, similar to menstruation, which occurs after stopping progestogen medication.

Wolff's Law Physiologic law which states that bone elements rearrange themselves and grow smaller or larger in response to stress.

Work capacity A measure of an individual's ability to perform physical work.

Zinc A metal element found in trace amounts in human tissues, including bone.

Index